N1 Nutritional

Programming

N1 Nutritional Programming:

The Fundamentals of Nutritional Programming

By Phil Learney

N1 Nutritional Programming: The Fundamentals of nutritional programming
ISBN 978-0-97809931-61537
ISBN 978-0-97809931-61506

The ideas, concepts, and opinions expressed in N1 Nutritional Programming are intended to be used for educational purposes only. The book is sold with the understanding that the author and publisher are not rendering medical advice of any kind, nor is the book intended to replace medical or qualified nutritional advice, nor to diagnose, prescribe or treat any disease, condition, illness, or injury.

It is imperative that before beginning nutritional program, you receive full medical clearance from a licensed physician.

The Food and Drug Administration has not evaluated the statements contained on PhilLearney. com or within N1 Nutritional Programming.

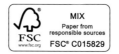

CONTENTS

Acknowledgments

I would first like to thank all the people that have believed in my instruction and guidance, especially those that prompted me to record them as a substantial piece of literature. I want to thank the people out there that believe in what I do those that travel distances, great or small, to hear me speak and those who log in daily to listen to my ramblings.

The support of my family has been invaluable. Even though they had their doubts when I stepped into this, at times, unforgiving career path, they have always been there. I am grateful to my dad, my sister, and my late mum, who I hope would have been proud of what I've achieved and that despite my slightly obscure choices in my educational journey I ended up doing something I love and am good at.

I want to thank my closest and greatest friends, those who I know I can always talk to or message, irrespective of the time between our last communication, and their unwavering understanding of my, often cluttered, mind that at times does get distracted. I love you all and you know who you are.

I'd like to give a big thank you to some people who have more directly supported what I've done:

Amy for your compulsive organization: without it, the time I would have had to write this book would have been considerably less. Not only the wife of one of my greatest friends, but also a great source of support.

Jose Antonio for being willing to give up some of his invaluable time and expertise to cast his critical eye over my work, undoubtedly at times cursing at my poor grasp of spelling and grammar. Apologies.

Heather Saunders for serving as my copyeditor and reviewing my entire manuscript with a fine-tooth comb to ensure it makes sense to all readers and rests easy on the eyes of those more adept at the English language than myself.

Nick for giving me the opportunity to remain in the U.K. and giving me a facility to serve as my base. Your support in all of my endeavors is hugely appreciated and never forgotten.

Finally, it wouldn't be right to exclude, given my personality, the doubters out there you fuel an ongoing fire and inherent need I have to prove points, so thank you for that.

PREFACE

I have worked in the health and fitness industry for nearly 20 years. In that time, I have coached over 14,000 hours of one-on-one sessions and worked with an array of clients from your everyday "Joe" to world-class international athletes. Throughout this time, I have developed many of my own opinions, methods, and practices all of which I have used, evaluated, adapted, and, in some cases, completely scrapped. I integrated information from others based on their sound logic, results, supporting science, and early in my career their authority.

More often than not, a specific system or method of practice will become popular and remain at the forefront of programming methodology for a time while it is studied and practically applied. This happens with programs focused on training, nutrition, and many aspects of physical health.

No matter its popularity or established nature, each program must be evaluated. I have personally found, through my own trial and error experiences (and trust me, there have been many), aspects that work and those that do not. Some practices needed to be adapted, whereas others were applicable for only a minority of clients. Some practices were only useful for short periods and then tapered off into no results or, worse, regression. Some practices achieved results, ranging from excellent to merely average.

With each session, I did my utmost to observe my clients, note each individual's progress, and maintain two-way communication. In doing so, I received a large amount of feedback pertaining to their emotions and compliance to the program. Conversely, if they were not compliant, I received feedback as to why not.

Reviewing client feedback and my experience, studying the commonalities and subtle differences, I reached conclusions that allowed me to make better and more effective decisions as a coach.

Over the years, I can conclusively say I know one thing to be true: we cannot, in our wildest dreams, fully control or understand the complexities of the human body. Whether we are talking about training or nutrition, we currently have nothing that will guarantee a specific outcome with all people at all times.

What we are left with is a catalog of ways to establish a starting point or point of reference. From this, with the ever-evolving and adapting organism that is the human body, we are left with what could be seen as perhaps the best practice, given both the present knowledge and experience of the coach, which is ultimately whatever works best for the individual.

Ever since the low-calorie, low-fat diets of old, every moment something new always arises and takes hold of the masses and dietary culture. As with fitness programs, some of these trends last the duration and some do not. Some adhere to scientific principles, whereas others are disputed from inception. Our role is to look critically at both the pros and cons of such programs with an unbiased, and skeptical, view. Paradigm shifts in science inevitably occur as we have more and more research at our disposal. What is considered fact now may be dismissed tomorrow.

We have much at our disposal that can influence our decisions. The prevailing power, however, in today's society comes from authority. Even now, you might be processing information in this preface based on my authority. I must ask you not to; rather, study the information provided here and then evaluate it research it, test it, and determine how it applies to you and your practices.

In this work, I provide both my experience and current scientific knowledge in the field. There will be points that you may disagree with or dispute. There may be points where my hold on current information is perhaps not as good as your own. But there will be many points that resonate and add value to your current programs. There will be many facts to help you expand your knowledge and grow as a coach.

I have put together this comprehensive guide to provide insight into the thought processes and reasoning behind many nutritional protocols and practices. It is not a complete reference, but rather a starting point and supplements work with a high-quality nutritional coach. This book will increase your awareness of factors that influence your decisions, your knowledge of the psychology and physiology behind your decisions, and your ability to learn from the outcomes of those decisions. From this book, you will develop a better understanding of what occurs during prescriptive nutritional programming and the numerous factors that influence you or your clients' lifestyle and physical development.

Chapter 1: Understanding Physical Change

The human being is an outstanding creature. From the moment of conception, we are constantly changing and adapting to our environment. It is not until many years later that we are able to influence our own personal environment and respond to it.

To understand physical change, we must first grasp what causes it and why we make some choices over others. To this day, many of us still make illogical choices based in habitual behaviors that have been positively reinforced by the people and environments around us. In many cases, this is simply a choice that has been made, drawn from our own conclusions or those of our closest peers.

These choices are often simple things that, in hindsight, we undoubtedly ask, "Why did I do that?" However, if we apply the same question preemptively, it puts us in the position to pursue the positive physiological outcome we seek.

> *"Insanity: doing the same thing over and over again and expecting different results."*
>
> *- Albert Einstein*

To elicit change, we must therefore make changes. Moreover, we must be willing and prepared to modify our outlook and therefore behavior. Nearly all of us have an inherent fear of this change. When allowed to, we will revert to our own tried and true methods, even if the outcome is suboptimal. When seeking to go beyond what has preceded us, there must be not only an openness to change, but also an outlook as free of bias as possible. The advanced nutritional methods we discuss typically derived from individuals or small groups that followed, often with no real understanding as to why, what was perhaps a diverse school of thought. These people only knew that this specific method was successful for them.

We must embrace that, in the pursuit of change, the process and design must be based on a desired and very specific outcome. What may be seen as a negative physiological outcome for one person may be positive for another. Clarification of the specific desired outcome at the onset remains critical in planning and executing an efficient and effective strategy. The uninformed assumption that everyone wants to be bigger and unfeasibly lean plagues our industry.

The metamorphosis of the human body cannot be viewed entirely as a scientific pursuit. Science, as useful and as credible as it is, still leaves us with many unanswered questions and inconclusive answers. We have what it gives us now and, beyond that, it is still in its infancy. The structure of the human body permits us to study it only from a gross anatomical and physiological perspective and leaves us again with more unanswered questions. Scientific studies allow us to conclude what is a best practice in small, sometimes randomized, and often specific populations. Collation of this data over the years may change our thinking or views on a specific practice, but does not detract from what coaches can see in front of them.

Understanding why something occurs leads us to better conclusions and more efficient, sustainable, and ultimately better outcomes. To disregard science would indeed be incredibly foolish, but to be led purely by its conclusions especially for an ever-evolving, diverse, and efficient organism would be equally as foolish. Science is part of a myriad of tools we must embrace to become better coaches and educators. Coaches who study the hierarchy of knowledge and consider science, logic, trial and error, authority, and tradition together are ultimately able to serve their clients better.

HUMAN DIFFERENTIALS

Every organism has an inherent variability and many components within it. Understanding what drives these components in the most efficient way helps us understand the morphological position or stage of development that individual might be in at that particular time. The fundamental basis of this is exactly what we are striving to understand and, in response, help influence. Not just on a physiological, psychological, and behavioral level, but alongside the other contributing facets of life and development. Understanding, or at least attempting to understand, individual traits that may have been inherited, those that may be congenital, and those acquired throughout an individual's lifespan leads us to a better understanding of the organism and its individual characteristics.

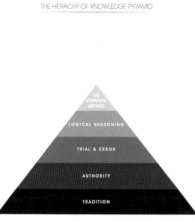

THE HIERARCHY OF KNOWLEDGE

Figure 1 The hierarchy of knowledge pyramid encompasses the ways we gather knowledge

During assessment, attributes such as height, body mass, muscle fiber type, hormonal makeup, neural capacity, and countless others must be considered. The nutritional methods used for physical advancement should only be developed following an in-depth analysis of an individual and a substantial body of evidence compiled from that analysis. Nutrition in itself is an applied form of biochemistry; therefore, we must have a rudimentary understanding of biochemistry itself, alongside the physiology of exercise, to apply it appropriately and with a solid basis.

Universal prescriptive methods and generic commercialized systems work on the principle that they have a reasonable chance of success within the context of a large participant group. Within these loose guidelines, there will inevitably always be a success story or two that continues to drive, promote, or popularize that particular method. Human nature lends us to talk about success openly, yet quietly blame failure on our own shortcomings. A successful media or viral campaign is all it takes in the modern world to solidify a method.

In the case of nutrition, success is often gauged by the slightly skewed bodyweight parameter (the number most people endeavor to reduce). Understanding the stages and factors involved in adaptation allows the coach to observe, analyze, and evaluate the individual with greater success. The greater the spectrum of tools we have for analysis, the more we can explain and rationalize our decisions, which will inevitably lead to better outcomes.

Something as simple as misunderstanding the direction behind your efforts or programming can ultimately lead to failure. Our goal is largely to minimize this risk by using available hierarchical evidence.

MANAGING HABITS AND BEHAVIOR

Let me be clear: you are responsible for changing people's nutritional habits. As coaches, we have a great responsibility: we are creating and forming new nutritional habits for our clients. Like most habits, if they are not monitored and integrated appropriately, they could develop negatively. In our case, this could mean unhealthy relationships with food.

Most certainly, the desire to eat nutritiously and avoid excessive amounts of processed and manufactured foods is not a bad thing. The problem in dividing our thoughts into eating "clean" or "dirty" is that it leads us to an excessive amount of either rigidity or a psychological approach that lacks care and concern for our well-being.

Many dietary approaches alter a person's physical and mental landscape. It is our responsibility as coaches to ensure this is not compounded into a long-term problem or a fixed and rigid mindset. Strategies need to be implemented at all times to avoid negatively altering a person's relationship with both their physical selves and food.

Much like any eating disorder, orthorexia (although currently not clinically seen as a mental or psychiatric condition) is an environment many coaches are unintentionally positioning people in. Over time, by omitting entire food groups or single foods without adequate or misplaced rationale, a fear over the ingestion of the aforementioned foods develops. Only in the case of severe allergens would fear serve any rational purpose.

It is our role to educate and emphasize throughout any given strategy why, at any particular stage, something may be absent, omitted, or replaced. Studies have supported the hypothesis that behavioral outcomes are largely compounded by the level of dietary restraint and rigidity. Adverse behaviors, such as binge eating, calorie counting, and the simple conscious process of dieting as we know it, all correlate to overeating and increases in body mass.[1,2]

Omitting any macronutrients or essential food groups for the long term combined with a "diet" or restrictive mentality yields a potential lack of nutrients, poor health, and possibly psychological challenges with food as a whole. We must avoid these scenarios at all cost. The general media exacerbates the problem, as do people on social media claiming to be authorities. Research tells us that a large percentage of those with disordered eating patterns also show classic signs of anxiety and obsessive-compulsive disorders (OCD).[3,6] The notion that the human body is capable of self-regulation and control is one that has also been lost amongst the dieting era and the large-scale processing of food.

> "In the world of dieting, particularly contest dieting, we must beg the question if the prevalence or a degree of OCD is, in fact, a necessity to success in itself."
> ~Phil Learney: The Science of Contest Prep 2014

It is our job as coaches to ensure education is prevalent at all times throughout any dietary process and to make sure the selective changes within this process are understood as temporary and merely serving a temporary purpose. The backlash from "dieting" in any of its extreme forms must be managed to guide the client's mindset and to avoid any negative behavioral outcomes.

Ultimately, our goal is to help put people in a position where there is both a healthy relationship with food and positive choices that provide feelings of well-being, satisfaction, and progression within their physical selves. These things must be carefully monitored throughout the process. Often, however, the urgency for results creates a negative situation. The responsible actions of advisors will ensure these are kept to the very minimum, given the constraints they are allowed to work in. In almost all cases, long-term sustainability, management, and progression are large parts of what is required.

Food must be understood for what it is. There is a distinct lack of evidence to indicate or corroborate the speculative notion that specific macronutrients or types of food show any addictive quality. The proponents of food "addiction" seem to disregard behavior, the thing we as coaches are most responsible for influencing.

The transformation-style diets so prevalent now require people to adhere to a restrictive regimen for perhaps 8–12 weeks that draws them away from everything they are used to and perhaps takes the enjoyment out of their diet. Upon completion, it is not addiction that makes them move into uncontrollable bouts of eating, but the restrictive pressure that has just been released from what was a short-term target (and one that lacks any form of sustainable patterning).[1,2]

I want to note here that most coaching businesses complain about the lack of long-term clients and income. However, they are repeatedly marketing time-restrictive, transformation-style programs that, at their conclusion, do not leave clients in their right mind or with a competitive goal they are likely to continue. The premise that food is addictive is flawed and dated.

Indeed, the psychological aspects and their association with behavior are of more interest.[7] Certain foods and food types do influence the reward center of the brain, particularly dopamine. Recent comparisons between class A drugs and sugar have been flaunted as rationale for the obesity epidemic. But these are missing the point this is an area of the brain stimulated through many things besides refined sugar.

Further, the fact that more of these "pleasurable" foods are available in today's society lacks any real substance as a correlation to obesity. The "quick fix" attitude we now have toward a lot of life, paired with the food industry's willingness to design and manufacture food that stimulates this pleasure response, is a two-way situation.[8] In the case of physical development, the willingness to change will almost always remain a more veracious drive, provided "reward" becomes part of the process and the plan is not entirely devoid of pleasure.

The psychological aspect of proverbially "falling off the wagon" can be seen as something imposed a restriction or a demand on an individual that was incorrectly managed. Palatability of food, variety, and reward must be integrated into an all-encompassing and ongoing approach. Those with issues that are more habitual may initially need mental diversion tactics to shift their focus in a different direction. The fact is, a particularly overweight person in the onset will undoubtedly require more discipline, as their habits and behavior are more ingrained and disruptive to both their health and physique. By default, though, these are the people that will often see fast physical changes, thus somewhat offsetting the reward and pleasure previously achieved through food.

Now, this is all completely reliant on an individualized, manageable, and sustainable approach. A client with a diet that you could grade with a 30% mark simply needs 35% to see progress. Many coaches immediately shoot for a 100% mark.

Much like you would not just throw 100 kg (~220 lbs.) on the back of someone who had never squatted more than 30 kg (~66 lbs.) in training, the stimulus must be progressive and analyzed throughout and then refined based upon response, mechanical considerations, and weak points in a supporting chain. Nutrition is no different. Ask for an extra 5 kg (~11 lbs.) on their backs first; when they achieve that, increase it.

Establishing homeostatic control by managing energetic or caloric factors is adequate for most coaches to start to positively manage the person's environment. We must realize inhibited eating will, in almost all cases, develop into disinhibited eating patterns and episodic binges.[1,2, 9–11] There are countless facets to food intake stress, anxiety, socioeconomic status but almost all appear to center around reward and pleasure.[12–15]

Not only is the way you handle your clients going to evolve, but so will the way you treat them to maintain the same ongoing success. We are fundamentally sales people. We are marketing concepts and changes in lifestyle that must beappealing, rewarding, and have both life-long and positive connotations for the client.

Ethically, we must fully understand the varied and evolving concepts to embrace the potential negative impact alongside the positive. An action creates a reaction and a reaction creates a by-product. Knowledge surrounding the actions, reactions, and by-products is all-encompassing. Most coaches market their wares by simply knowing the reaction, the potential reaction, or indeed their own reaction to a given stimulus.

Thankfully, the approaches of modern coaches are becoming not only more effective and efficient, but shrouded in more ethical and moral decisions pertaining to their client's physical and mental well-being. This only serves to positively support what we do. Helping a client achieve rapid weight loss is not sustainable, but is a huge selling point. Allowing an overweight client inordinate amounts of flexibility in their approach will often initially yield suboptimal results but better sustainability. We must be adept in the balancing act between rigidity and flexibility and, as previously mentioned, the psychological and behavioral management that overlays them.

Keeping a client is not only about business, but also often about the fact that many people are still on their journey. They need to persist and continue to progress in all facets of their physical and emotional development, but alongside that, they need to continue to be educated.

Remember, we are teaching people to manage these things themselves, and empowering them to make decisions to sustain what they achieve.

COMPLIANCE

Ask any coach in any modality and they will more than likely concur that compliance is the biggest factor in the success or failure of any plan or formula. We can look at this very narrowly and ascertain that this is simply up to the clients' character, as well as how much they want or value their goals. As we progress, we will learn that compliance is not simply achieved through a coach's ability to motivate or inspire, but concomitantly through their understanding of how the human body adapts and regulates function under situations of stress.

If we look at the narrow perspective and ascertain that compliance is compounded largely by how much you value the outcome and your goals, these goals must be clear to you and your client at all times. As coaches, we are often asked many questions we must deliberate over:

- Does walking around with abs year-round supersede being able to socialize with friends without creating undue emotional and mental

- Do you and your client have strength and determination in achieving your tasks and goals?
- How do you deal with the non-conformity that will inevitably occur?
- Once that resolve is undermined, will that temporal release from your "diet" lead to you make the most of the indulgence and continue until a new threshold or day begins?
- Do you accept the indulgence as merely a choice, as opposed to a failure?
- How does your client regard food: is food perceived or identified as "bad" or "good?"

Some of these questions will be answered as these issues occur or feedback is received regarding a period embarking upon something new. Each leads us to more intelligent deductions surrounding non-conformity and leads us away from the basic notion that it is a lack of cognitive inhibition (willpower) or the client "wanting" their goals enough. There are more in-depth psychological and physiological mechanisms at play that I hope, upon the conclusion of this text, you understand far more about.

This is comparable to making mistakes in life. Does that mistake resonate in your head or do you just move on and see it as a moment in which you learned something? Can this be overcome with an approach that allows what could be seen as a mistake to also be seen as merely a learning curve?

To tap into the psyche of a human being is fascinating and to see someone succeed against adversity and inordinate challenges is what drives me, and many others, to do what I do. There will be emotional and physiological barriers in our way that will test both the coach and client.

The psychology of behavior and associations with the temporal satisfaction that, for many, dietary indulgence will resolve, will always stand in our way. A phrase I despise, but seems relevant right now, is that moderation is actually key to what we strive for.

The dominant factor that drives the yo-yo dieting culture is largely behavioral and psychological. This is underpinned by the metabolic adaptations or adaptive thermogenesis that comes with common dietary practices used by coaches and the dieting public. An intelligent coach will attempt to attenuate negative behavioral and psychological patterning, thus positively affecting and supporting thermogenesis.

A large part of what we do is supporting and encouraging people in addition to the all-important coaching. Ensuring support networks are in place can aid in this. Friends, family, and those you surround yourself with will tell you to see it through. In doing so, the by-product of this action is the filtering of who is truly supportive and who is not. Remember that you are asking those around you to also embrace your change.

For some, this will be incomprehensible and the changes to your lifestyle that you had in common with them will often irreparably be questioned. This can be a hard process for many. Another human trait is acceptance and being different remains frowned upon in society. The older we become, the more ingrained habits and behavior also inevitably become. This is often reflective of the people we have surrounded ourselves with. So, when embarking upon such a major shift in lifestyle, choose to position those with closer behavioral and psychological traits around you.

"If all else fails, I always think proving doubters wrong is a pretty strong incentive for anything in life."
~Phil Learney: Advanced Nutritional Strategies 2015

INITIAL ASSESSMENT OF A CLIENT

From initial contact, it is critical that the process of gathering information pertaining to your client has begun. This will make your decision-making process with both training and nutrition easier and likely more successful. From the initial conversation, you can be gathering valuable information that will help support client compliance and ensure a successful outcome to the process.

How we gather this information is never-ending. Our senses become a tool: our observation, our communication, and our feedback. Noting the potentially compromised circulation upon shaking your client's hand can direct a line of questioning and is a clue that alone is flimsy and irrelevant, but considered cumulatively with other clues can direct our efforts better.

THE STAGES OF ADAPTATION

The principle of adaptation is quite simply an organism's ability to adjust to its environment. This phenomenon is something that can occur in seconds in the lifespan of a single organism or bridge generations of an entire species. Through intricate planning and execution of nutritional stimuli, we are capable of altering and molding an organism in this case, the human body in a specific way.

For those seeking aesthetic improvements, results hinge on this specificity. When considering the human body, it must be clearly understood that a single rule cannot and probably never will apply. Coaches out there claiming to have the best, or most effective, program for a given adaptive response simply have one that, through intricate planning or merely chance, will elicit a suitable amount of success in some cases, sufficient for enough impressive changes to continue to market it as an all-encompassing solution. It is not, however, a license to stroke their ego or take advantage of those who, through desperation, are willing to try anything. Anyone can tout a system or sell a short-lived concept and perhaps even spend their life moving from fad to fad.

But the truly successful coaches will embrace conceptual program design, customize it, and apply it at the correct time and stage of a person's physiological and life development. When looking at systems and methodology, we must be prepared to understand and embrace both their inherent flaws and noted benefits before we can make an educated decision as to their application and validity of use. Too many systems are flaunted by many as the way to do something, which only serves to solidify the coaches' lack of physiological understanding and their necessity to become part of a collective unimpressionable way of thinking. Remember, a good coach must have an open mind.

"It does take great maturity to understand that the opinion we are arguing for is merely the hypothesis we favor, necessarily imperfect, probably transitory, which only very limited minds can declare to be a certainty or a truth."
~Milan Kundera

Often, when determining which stimulus is the best, it is not just the value we must consider, but the cost as well. It all becomes a series of trade-offs, much like in the biological states of anabolism and catabolism: without both existing, we cannot adapt, yet each has a concurrent cost.

Through understanding and experience, the cost of these trade-offs becomes less and less due to the coach's level of expertise and level of subconscious intuition. You cannot teach this experience and cannot always rely on science as our sole method of decision-making. We must, at all times, assess and correct our methods of adaptation to prevent stagnation, and evolve nutritional practices as the body changes and alters the way it manages metabolic processes.

For these reasons, the defining characteristics of nutritional programs must revolve around carefully considered parameters. Lack of consideration for the individual means we are crunching numbers and considering only superficial information. Planning a nutritional strategy around a formula, or a training routine around textbook data, shows the lack of experience, flaws, or simple laziness in a coach's approach to their client.

Plans simply become the consumption of nutrients in a different or methodical way. Differentiating between a true "nutritional" program and a diet is what defines results. Without careful consideration of genotype, phenotype, and demand-based and biological factors, we are merely left with a generic template of requirements and the assumption that the human body will simply adapt accordingly, and in the way we hope.

Failure on all these fronts will result in the profit of the adaptation being offset by the cost. Looking simply at the basic "more (or less) is better" mentality of most, the balancing act between stimulus and adaptation is often lost. This is not to say that the end physical goal is not achievable far from it. But, in the grander scheme of things, we are also looking at the aforementioned cost, which encompasses not only the physiological changes, but also the behavioral and psychological implications.

Despite physiological outcomes being largely predictable, the human body is too efficient an organism to be tied down with purely textbook practices. Though an anatomy text tells us the details of what our systems are made up of, it merely touches upon how one thing can lead to thousands, potentially millions, of cascade effects across the body's internal systems.

Our ability as coaches to use basic principles and science alongside our professional experience defines our individual methodology and intervention. A qualitative analysis of the individual and an educated decision-making process are required at all times. The one-size-fits-all approach merely bottlenecks our knowledge and leads to confirmation bias.

CHAPTER 2: THE CONSEQUENCE OF CHANGE

Adjusting any habit causes stress to the body above its usual level. The response to this stress comes in the form of systemic overcompensation and the corresponding physiological adjustment. The body is a self-regulating organism that, at all times, is altering cascades of hormones and physiological mechanisms in an attempt to maintain a level of survival.

This basic principle relies heavily on a multitude of intrinsic and extrinsic factors but must always be considered a fundamental principle to positive adaptation and a requirement in the pursuit of lean muscular gain, fat loss, or performance enhancement.

The concept of periodization in training is based around Selye's general adaptation syndrome and looks at the effect of accumulating stress in detail. This exact same principle, in many respects, can be applied to nutrition. The similarities in advanced nutritional methodology and training periodization are not that dissimilar.

It must be noted when planning any nutritional program that change itself is a form of stress and the management of stress is part of the myriad of challenges we coaches face. Nutritional change is likely the most important, yet the most detrimental when miscalculated.

The human organism is a mass of physiological potential. When confronted with a perceived threat, it reacts with a pronounced stress response. In addition to this implications should our calculations be in gross error.[16]

PHYSIOLOGICAL AND PSYCHOLOGICAL STRESS

The idea that the destruction of something will lead to it organically replenishing itself sounds like something from a science fiction movie, right? On a daily basis, those of you that elicit a calculated stimulus and trauma on the body, and then correspondingly and intelligently nourish it, are doing exactly that.

Further, you are specifically adapting to the nature of the destruction and adjusting to prevent reoccurrence. Pretty incredible, isn't it? It is like tiny little controlled pockets of evolution. This is one of the things that excites me the most about what we do as coaches the ability of the human body to change and adapt to its environment and our ability to influence that.

If we consider the basics of the human body, we know it is constantly trying to live in a state of equilibrium (homeostasis). On one side of homeostasis, we have a state of cellular destruction (catabolism catabolic, destructive metabolism) and on the other, a state of cellular regeneration (anabolism anabolic, constructive metabolism). A catabolic state is a state of survival a state in which the endocrine system senses danger and responds accordingly. An anabolic state is a state of regeneration and recovery. Both states complement each other and are essential for physical adaptation and development.

It is at this stage we come across a predicament. We rely heavily on stress hormones, part of the catabolic state, if we are to control destruction and the breaking down of the body through training. If uncontrolled, this can lead to widespread tissue destruction, muscle loss, bone degeneration, immune suppression, and even neural destruction. This also affects fat loss and compositional changes. In a catabolic state, the body will potentially use fat mass and fat-free mass (FFM, or lean tissue). Our goal is to minimize the trade-off by revising the duration we spend in each state. We will discuss this in detail later in the text.

HOW DOES STRESS AFFECT US?

Stress can be extrinsic or intrinsic and its origins can stem from many areas: stresses can be personal, physical, mental, toxic, or chemical. The interesting thing is the physiological reactions and responses are very similar for all types of stress.[16]

SELYE'S GENERAL ADAPTATION SYNDROME

Based on his research on stress, endocrinologist Hans Selye believed there were three distinct reactions exhibited by humans in response to stress, regardless of the nature of the stressor, which could be physical, emotional, or environmental. Based on this premise, he developed the general adaptation syndrome, which has three stages.[17–19]

ALARM REACTION

The first stage is the alarm reaction, which occurs when we are surprised or threatened. This can be encountered acutely through a training stimulus or by using stimulants that influence the nervous system. This can also be encountered in much lower and more chronic levels by an ongoing or acute caloric deficit and concurrent state of physiological survival.

Through a sympathetic reaction, our adrenaline levels rise, causing an elevation above our body's natural homeostasis. This stage initiates the fight-or-flight response and correspondingly focuses on the immediate muscular and emotional requirements to either confront or flee from the stressor. This reaction addresses the immediate requirements, but suppresses non-essential functions, such as the digestive system.

If the alarm reaction is caused by an injury, there is an increase in whole-body protein loss, mainly from myofibrillar muscle proteins. Throughout the stages of the general adaptation syndrome, there is evidence that nutritional, hormonal, and pharmacologic support prevents destructive metabolic processes (catabolism).[20]

STAGE OF RESISTANCE

The second stage tasks the body with finding ways to cope with the stress if it persists. These mechanisms signal the adrenal glands to release hormones: cortisol, growth hormone (GH), and norepinephrine.

Cortisol diverts glucose for use by the brain, while allowing amino and fatty acids to be used for energy. Norepinephrine works part and parcel with cortisol, and is part of the catecholamine group that will affect heart rate, assist in the release of glucose, and increase muscular blood flow and oxygen supply to the brain.

Now consider uncontrolled stress. When we step in the weight room, this stress is controlled and, for the most part, regulated. We target physical stress to prompt specific responses, while providing the body with the nutrients it requires pre- and post-workout to elicit this response safely and efficiently, and to help the body recover from it.

The problem we have is that modern life puts us in a position where the spikes in cortisol and other stress hormones are frequent and, in some cases, chronic with no corresponding bout of physical exertion or control. Compound this with general day-to-day life and these cascading hormones are generally spiraling out of control and can become chronically high. If we were to impose restrictive barriers surrounding food intake, the entire stress response would become exacerbated.

The chronic elevation of these stress hormones can disrupt carbohydrate metabolism, cholesterol levels, and management of cardiovascular systems. They may also cause premature aging and are implicated as a major contributor to obesity, insomnia, heart disease, digestive problems, depression, and memory impairment.[21, 22]

Excessive amounts of processed foods in a person's diet in both frequency and magnitude deplete critical nutrients over time and increase nervous system reactivity, irritability, nervousness, and deplete the reserves that enable adequate recovery from these bouts of stress. Prolonged poor dietary habits and the resultant lowered concentrations of key nutrients in the blood can impair brain function. Studies have also suggested that chronic stress, unlike acute stress,[23] may affect the amount of orexigenic or feeding peptides. Acute stress tends to increase anorexigenic peptides (one of the reasons why post-workout, people often have no appetite). This could also suggest that the level of satiety post-workout may be an indicator of the level of chronic or acute stress.

> "Appetite is controlled by a distinct neuronal circuitry consisting of an interconnected network of pathways that contain both orexigenic (increasing food intake) and anorexigenic (decreasing food intake) signals."
>
> Samantha Chagra[24]

After the stressor is gone, the parasympathetic system led by the hypothalamus takes over and reverses the impact of the sympathetic response by slowing the heart rate and respiration back to normal levels, relaxing the muscles, and starting non-essential functions. The resting point comes when the body finds homeostasis. In terms of nutrition, this would be when anabolism and catabolism are physiologically matched an impossible scenario.

This is one of many reasons the traditionally restrictive caloric and macronutrient models fail for people with a history of poor eating habits and chronic stressors. With these models, focus remains purely on physical change without the necessary psychological and behavioral adaptations. Stressors, for the most part, lie outside of dietary choices. The habitual changes and extreme restrictions posed by many dietary approaches create negative connotations and an increase in anxiety disorders and obsessive tendencies now associated with these eating habits. We will discuss food and food choices in more detail in later chapters; however, we should always revert to the simple notion that dietary practices that can be adhered to, that correspond with the client's current lifestyle, and that progress toward the desired outcome are what we strive for.

Restricting food is like a wall with a sign that reads "No Graffiti:" the wall is typically covered by spray paint, whereas the adjoining walls are not. It is the same with dietary restrictions: if we impose a restriction on someone, we challenge their psyche. The second that psyche is broken, so are the floodgates.

Creating a rationale behind any imposed restriction is like telling the graffiti artist they will get access to the wall, just not this second; and when they do finally get access, they will approach the wall with a greater palette of paint. Nutrition is about education, alongside the coaching of modulatory patterns and habits far above and beyond any imposed restrictions, which is how "diets" are generally viewed.

STATE OF EXHAUSTION

The final stage occurs when the stage of resistance is poorly managed. The body's resources at this point are close to, or beyond, an exhaustive state, with the duration and/or level of stress surpassing what the body can physiologically cope with. This affects what has been termed the "adaptive reserve." Recovery from this state, for many, will not only result in better overall health and compositional improvements, but a strong and efficient immune system.

Let's return to exercise and its largely non-structured nature, in comparison to the more structured concept of training. Tie this in with the classical thought of "less is better" concerning energetic intake and the widely accepted notion that "more is better" concerning exercise or training and we stumble upon an issue.

This approach immediately predisposes us to an excessive level of physiological stressors that are potentially manageable in the short term, but are detrimental in the long term. This pushes our regenerative reserves to the limit and therefore potentially moves us into a chronic state of degeneration. The challenge we face when attempting to debunk this theory is that, in the short term, it will meet the participant's desired and primary goal of "weight" loss.

This is perhaps one of the reasons we see people repeating this same cyclical methodology to no avail. Over and over again, they achieve only a level of short-term success with inevitable overall long-term failure. Perhaps we look to the short-term pleasure of things far too much as a population, instead of considering the long term.

Undoubtedly, these approaches play to positive psychology because, at the outset, they may support and move toward the participant's goal. This leads to continuing support for the approach and, sometimes, viral popularization. People do not just want a platform in which to shout from; they also want to feel part of something.

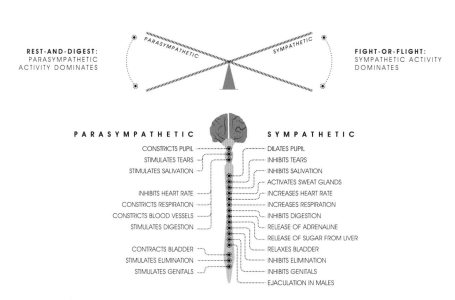

Figure 2 Homeostasis and the SNS and PSNS. Homeostasis is a balance between the rest-and-digest actions of the PSNS and the fight-or-flight actions of the SNS.

Over time in almost all of these methods, participant enthusiasm and compliance will no doubt falter as they move into the longer term. At this point, it is almost inevitable they will blame themselves either consciously or subconsciously for their failings, as opposed to the shortcomings of the actual system they opted to follow. After all, who wants to act as an ambassador for something with great excitement and passion only to then fall on their face when it fails? Often, people will accept the failure as their own, rather than blame the flawed system or methodology.

These cycles then, in time, often repeat themselves. After the individuals stop pursuing their original goal, they simply recollect the short-term results they achieved. Then, when that day arrives that a little weight needs shifted, they once again revert to what previously worked, often paying both physically and financially for the privilege.

In life, people will run up financial debt to obtain what they desire in that particular moment. This is as true in finance as it is in physiological goals. Getting into that dress, looking better for a holiday people will use all manner of short-term and extreme methodology to lose what may only accumulate to a few pounds of weight. The physical difference we would see from this is almost negligible, but how it makes people psychologically feel about themselves could become quite profound. However, these short-term aggressive approaches do come at a cost, much like the interest on a credit card.

Again, people deal with the debt or cost it incurs when required to, as opposed to preventing the "pain" element of it in the present.

One of our jobs as coaches is to ensure the cost of any approach is both understood and managed while ensuring goals are simultaneously achieved and ideally maintained. Anyone can elicit weight loss even fat loss, if there is adequate trust in the coach and compliance by the client. The belief that what many are advising is correct (often why people ask those that have achieved visible success how they did it) and that the person asking the questions is prepared to actually change something long term or simply for a given period.

Individuals who are losing or have lost weight often are granted authority on the subject, if not through their own beliefs, but that of their peers. They are often seen as those who perhaps have a "secret" to share. In many cases, these people are ill qualified to give advice. Many may have issues, perhaps both physiologically and psychologically, toward both their management and relationship with food and exercise. Many followed something they poorly understand why or how it worked; they just simply know the mechanics of it, so to speak.

Much like young men resonate toward the biggest guy in the gym for advice, many people are drawn to the appearance of a successful plan. They do not understand that their journey might be different and whatever someone else did before becomes praised as the magic formula. This also occurs heavily with coaches who take what works for them, with a poor understanding of the program's intricacies, and then replicate it across their clientele. Given the differentials discussed earlier, we can see why this is often a bad approach.

Losing weight, much like building muscle tissue or developing a six-pack, does not justify authority in a matter pertaining to science, formal education, and the all-important inclusion of practical experience. A swift look through your social networking news feed should serve well to dismiss that notion.

Seeking advice from someone based on the fact they "look like they know what they are doing" is tantamount to me smearing grease on my hands, throwing on a pair of overalls and telling Lewis Hamilton that I can fix his Formula 1 car. Remind your coaches to educate themselves beyond their own personal experiences.

The body, in many respects, is quite simple; counteract stress and bouts of physical exertion with adequate recovery and restoration. The more stress the body is put under, the more emphasis must be placed on recovery and restoration. Removing as many stressors as possible is tantamount to success, particularly in elite athleticism the area we see recovery techniques often embraced. The general population would undoubtedly benefit from the removal or reduction of controllable stressors alongside the use of recovery and restoration methods. Our focus in this area for the purposes of this book is nutrition and endocrine support.

CONSIDERING ADAPTIVE RESERVE

Adaptive reserve is the term often coined for the substrates and energy reserve available for adaptation and recovery, as the name may suggest. Because the human body is dynamic by nature, this level of adaptive reserve is constantly in flux. Through careful planning and communication, we can determine if this becomes compromised and, through trial and error with our clientele, understand what may perhaps be too much or inadequate stimulus or stress for them as individuals.

Adaptive reserve is spread across an individual's requirements and demands. For example, if we use weight training as a basic method, a client looking to increase muscular size as their primary goal must consider that anything outside of this focus will diminish the adaptive reserve used for this job. This is not a negative thing, as for many, their desires to be better across the board at many aspects of fitness are not at the extremes of given spectrums: they do not have to be catwalk models or pro bodybuilders.

However, it will compromise a goal if substrates are not managed according to demands inclusive of energy systems. In this particular example, if glycogen is being diminished from distance running, the substrate available for muscle building is not only diminished, but the specific stimulus of weight training is now adapting to the need to carry bodyweight over long distances. You see where the issue lies. That is not to say it is an impossible feat, but the requirement of nutritional and endocrine substrates would be enormous and with the exception of someone genetically gifted, hormonally assisted, or with a capacity to handle large amounts of nutrients practically impossible.

Determining a client's primary goal and their willing trade-offs paints us a better picture of what is achievable in what timeline. This trade-off may often be what they have historically enjoyed or what they might enjoy under the idea it will bring them closer to their goals.

Adaptive reserve has its links with both genotype and phenotype. The "potential" that someone has will be often derived from this capacity. It will most certainly play a large factor at an elite level of almost any sport. Putting your training efforts into the reserves you adapt most efficiently to, or have a larger capacity for, would be the wisest approach. This, however, does not limit someone from wishing to do something against the grain, as such. It just means they may not excel at it. Nutrition permits us to nourish a system in the hope of supporting it. Considering energetic demands alongside macronutrient requirements is something often overlooked when considering performance and the adaptation of the body.

Consider that performance of a client often lies as one of the trade-offs to fat loss. You are putting them in a caloric deficit through either reduction in caloric intake or an increase in output. Demands, therefore, outweigh an individual's capacity to recover effectively. This is how we go about breaking the body's stores down if fat loss is the goal, this state is unavoidable. Remaining in such a state for extended periods of time will therefore diminish substrate reserves and eventually the body will begin to falter. Injury, sickness, and the inevitable metabolic adaptations that slow both weight and fat loss down will occur.

Adaptive reserve must be considered with an individual's current lifestyle. I recall when the stock market crashed; I took the frequency of training down for several of my clients who were emotionally impacted by it. It was a simple management of stressors, but I assure you, they appreciated it. People returning to training following a more "social" weekend may perhaps need their training adjusted accordingly, as you know their adaptive reserve has potentially been compromised. At the trade-off of an infrequent and diverse movement away from their normal life, they relaxed, de-stressed mentally, and enjoyed themselves. This is not inherently a bad thing, and can be okay in moderation, and for some it might even be a requirement psychologically. But the proportion of such events must still be in line with their goals. If the goal was to have fun and that was achieved it once again becomes simply a trade-off. Of value? That is a discussion between both coach and client.

Relaxation and the mental approach is a big part of sustainability and creating a better lifestyle (and physique) for most. It is essentially our job to monitor these variations in reserves and adapt accordingly. Proper training programming in conjunction with adequate nutrition and recovery are all keys to progress more stress, less recovery. One of the major quandaries we have at this stage is that some of the primary symptoms of stress, overtraining, and adrenal fatigue overlap. Unfortunately, failing to self-regulate makes the problem worse and can cause the following:

- Tiredness and a sense of sleepiness during the day
- Food cravings comfort and physiological requirements (elevation of orexigenic hormones)
- Needing stimulants or high doses of caffeine in coffee, energy drinks, or sodas
- Poor immune function
- Physical soreness and poor recovery
- Difficulty waking up and regulating energy levels
- Abrupt weight loss or weight gain

There are obvious ways in which to deal with this equation, but I rely on my experience and use a cross section of the population. We can assume that almost all of the populations we deal with as trainers are overstressed, many times undernourished, and many may be chasing a tail that will never be caught perhaps this stands true for ourselves.

The number of coaches I have had to pull the reins in on with training and up their dietary intake is unbelievable. The number of non-elite athletes that claim to be overtraining, again in my experience, are often simply under recovered.

> *"If you can improve recovery by 10% through restoration strategies and an improvement in nutrition, we can increase training stress by 10%. This gives us a performance improvement of 20%. The difference between a full-time professional athlete and a talented amateur is often far less than 20%. Ask yourself what you're prepared to give or do."*
>
> ~Phil Learney: Overtraining 2012

Therefore, you must consider lifestyle carefully and look at what creates stressors within it. A perfect scenario for physique development, would be one in which the release of stress hormones would be exclusively reserved for acute and goal-specific bouts of training and periods of excitement that accompany what we often define as "living," as opposed to the chronic dull level of stress that overshadows many of us on a daily basis.

This is not to say stress is by any means bad: the abundance of stress hormones is not only critical to our existence and adaptation, but a significant part of, quite literally, the excitement in our lives. We need them to build muscle and to burn fat. The goal is to avoid chronic overexposure. Become efficient. Try to pinpoint what exactly causes stress for you or your client external to your goals and pleasure. If you can, remove it or find a way to manage it better.

Minimize your exposure to stimuli you do not need. Reserve the heavy use of stimulants to "keep you going," for when you want to enjoy a good cup of coffee, or when you have a workout pending that is worthy of a little jolt prior to it. I will touch on caffeine more in chapters 7 and 9 regarding its properties and applicable use. Elevated stress hormones can positively assist training, but in the same breath can have the opposite effect. Acute elevation helps mobilize fatty acids through an intense focused exercise or training session and/or the use of exogenous stimulants such as caffeine. Overstimulation means we lose this acute positive impact and a resultant down-regulation of everything responsible. Over time, we fatigue important endocrine glands and create a cascade of negative adjustment throughout the entire body.

This does not just end here. Part of this process is to remove the emotional turmoil that may have inevitably come with overly restrictive dieting and repair the internal conflicts the body and mind go through when food is restricted or omitted for any length of time. For many people, the emotional stress that accompanies dieting far exceeds the physical stress. For this reason, their emotional attachments around food must be managed. More so than ever before, this is the largest factor I encounter that differs from as little as a decade ago.

"Food should not be seen or used as a reward. Research has shown us that using palatable foods as a reward makes them more appealing. The opposite occurs in that the alternative, healthy foods are then perceived as punishment."
~Puhl and Schwartz[25]

A study in Eating Behaviors in 2003 looked at the eating habits of 122 adults and their memories as children. Those that recollected the use of food as reward and/or punishment showed increased likelihood to use restrictive dieting and indulge in binge eating.[25] Once again, this is why we need to establish history alongside current habits and behavior.

Chapter 3: Physical Considerations

Many individuals lend themselves toward a sympathetic nervous system (SNS) that is sensitive to the impact of catecholamines (stress hormones).

When the SNS is overstimulated both acutely and chronically, it can lead to a loss of appetite and, in some cases, a disordered eating pattern similar to that of overweight or serial dieters. Despite the inherent flaws in his methodology, the system of psychosomatotypology proposed by Sheldon (discussed further in chapter 4) found what we commonly term "hard gainers," or ectomorphs, as those most likely to be highly sensitive to SNS stimulation.

These people also, in my experience, tend to be more introverted by nature. Commonly, yet not always, these individuals appear to generally show a higher tolerance to carbohydrates and higher overall thyroid output. The interactions with the SNS are apparent but not always conclusive. The complex link between the cascade of hormones that regulate the body and our eating patterns is merely in its infancy but is certainly worthy of consideration.

Principles to Consider

There are numerous principles we would consider when structuring a training regimen. These principles also largely apply to nutritional practices.

SPECIFICITY

The principle of specificity is quite simple. It implies that to improve at a particular exercise or skill one must perform that exercise or skill. The specificity training principle is referred to as "specific adaptation to imposed demands" (SAID).[27] In the context of nutrition, this is taking the history of someone's nutrition while considering their current physiological state.

From this, we are able to pinpoint systems that may have been excessively stimulated or under stimulated. By using a food log and cross correlating it with blood work, we are able, in an ideal scenario, to pinpoint nutritional deficiencies that then require a specific stimulus, replenishment, or stress alleviated from them. To be able to use alternative substrates as fuel, we must at times change both the supply and demand.

The role of a coach would be to spot the physiologically weak or strong point within a nutritional regimen and prescribe a change with respect to eradicating or balancing that indifference. This, in some cases, may call for the use of auxiliary nutrients (supplemental nutrition) to move or encourage a metabolic system to move forward or the short-term omittance of something to reinforce a habit or minimize nutritional stress. For example, if someone was overly dominant through the anterior head of the deltoids, you may omit direct work for a while before equilibrium is gained then, and only then, would you reintroduce specific work.

PROGRESSIVE OVERLOAD

The principle of overload and underload is looking at the energy and substrate levels required for the body relative to its imposed demands and requirements. We must endeavor to overload systems by moving into a caloric surplus, thus taking advantage of the anabolic state.

Alternatively, we must move into a caloric deficit (underload) to achieve the state of catabolism necessary for fat loss. With the two metabolic states anabolism (regeneration) and catabolism (degeneration) we must endeavor to make the metabolism work hard without "detraining" through any prolonged period of caloric restriction or surplus.

VARIETY

Nutrition by default should be varied. The slight variance foods give us allows our body to avoid stagnation and serves us a variety and mixture of nutrients at all time. In the world of overly restrictive and controlled dieting, there is often a lack of variance. Over time, this can impose larger than necessary demands on specific enzymes and catalysts to the breakdown of particular foods. This is part of the reason that when unnecessarily omitting certain foods or food types, upon returning to consumption, they create a reaction often bracketed as an allergy or intolerance.

People blame nutrients for all manner of reactions. The best example would be again carbohydrates and gluten. When someone is told they cannot eat something, it then becomes "forbidden fruit." For many, when they break from their rigid protocol and decide to consume something, they very rarely consume in a small amount. The floodgates open and they binge on large amounts of it. Someone who has an unfavorable reaction not an allergy or intolerance by any means, but maybe a small amount of bloating immediately blames the nutrient. They then revert to full omittance. Their body only knows the two extremes: nothing or enormous amounts.

Take note of this, as many self-diagnosed cases of food allergies and intolerances will be due to this. Small amounts of any food reintroduced strategically into people's diets allow the body to become accustomed or re-accustomed to it.

In the case of refined or processed foods that are often devoid of enzymes (to prevent rotting and enhance shelf life), the sheer abundance in many diets means they become imbalanced or devoid with what should be acquired from our actual diet.

Variety can simply be an alternative food, yielding similar macronutrients from a similar family. The different nutritional value, for example, in 30 grams of nuts across all varieties is often too little to even concern you, but the micronutrient variance is quite notable.

REVERSIBILITY

Everybody wants to look like a superhero (well, if you are reading this, you probably already do). Others simply wish they could feel better. They want to become leaner, stronger, lighter, heavier, more toned, and so on.

The specificity principle first helps us understand the need for and role of different nutritional methods and the impossibility of such a varied set of short-term goals. Pursuance of such a wide variance of goals would result in mastery of none, so it is critical we understand the primary and secondary goals of athletes, our clients, and ourselves.

Building muscle and losing fat are obviously metabolically associated, but the crossover only exists in the fact that each benefits from the other: building muscle helps lose fat and losing fat helps build muscle. Reversibility lends support to the basic biological principle of "if you do not use it, you lose it." Within a nutritional environment, the intelligent selection of a stimulus throughout any goal-oriented phase allows the components required for the primary goal to be kept at the forefront, whereas others are only momentarily and minimally compromised.

The art of nutritional cycling must be understood to reduce gross impairment of the secondary goal while remaining in pursuit of the primary goal. As mentioned, an example of this is the "bulking" approach, when muscular gain has been concurrently accepted alongside a level of fat gain. The extended and extreme period of hypercaloric dieting was accepted under the hope that when dieted down, some of it would remain. Through both science and experience, we know that this approach is, in many respects, counterproductive. Excessive and prolonged elevation of body fat serves no purpose to either goal and presents us with a series of trade-offs when we move into the aptly named cutting phase.

We can look to weight training and how many systems have evolved within that field. Conjugate periodization became popularized due to the detraining that occurred in the alternative block periodization methods. The conjugate system would look to integrate several modalities into a single training phase. Over the course of a week, perhaps the trainee would look to train for both speed and maximal strength. This would ensure that there was carry over from each modality. The progression would not be as dramatic as the block method (training for weeks at a time on a single modality), but clients saw less drop off in the other requisite. In this case, the idea would be to improve the force equation: Force = Mass x Acceleration.

In the case of nutrition, many approaches have moved away from the block methods of bulking and cutting to approaches in which both modalities are coached at the same time. Each complements the other: periods of bulking (hypercaloric) would be interspersed with cutting (hypocaloric) over shorter periods. Depending upon the weak point, more emphasis may be placed on the other. In training, someone may lack in acceleration but be able to move large masses; therefore, they would do a higher ratio of speed training in a training block. In nutrition, someone may lack muscle mass, but may hold little body fat. They would therefore use a higher ratio of hypercaloric dieting.

It must be noted that our adaptive response to certain nutrients and their corresponding impact on the endocrine system all have a differential lag time. Because of this fact, certain strategies can be acutely employed without the negative physiological connotations that are brought about and seen by more chronic dietary strategies.

Caloric deficits and surplus, fasting, flexible dieting, and hitting macros all have their place. Chronic overuse or incorrect application is when we encounter muted progress or, in some cases, regression. In the diet "industry," more often than not, the positive effects of these systems are noted and used as promotional tools to market, popularize, or promote such systems. The negative aspects, however, become selectively ignored. These are, for the most part, simple and effective business strategies to encourage the sale of products surrounding a system or the need to create a following to cement someone's involvement. People, even coaches, ultimately sell a generic or simple dietary dream.

Our goal is to establish progression without regression and use the tool most effective given the scenario, the physiological and psychological state of the individual, and their needs and wants.

Can we fast? Can we restrict calories? Can we obtain flexibility in food choices? Yes, we can. It is just a matter of determining when we can appropriately and most effectively apply them. Almost like a simple mathematical sum, can an individual's lifestyle, training, and nutrition work in synergy to elicit their desired outcome? Often the answer is no. This is where, as a coach, we need to advise as to the best equation to the three facets to elicit the best possible outcome given the circumstances. The single template many coaches adopt and feel ownership to only applies to a small number of people. Almost all popularized dietary systems hold some sway; it is our job to figure out which has the best and ultimately most sustainable outcome.

INDIVIDUALITY

The principle of individuality allows us to understand the basic premise that all humans are not created the same. In response to a stimulus, every individual will elicit an individual high or low response depending upon his or her genetics, environmental interactions, heredity, and a host of other factors.

Modern nutritional programs are often based upon the "least chance of failure" principle and the premise that as long as weight loss is achieved, nothing else fundamentally matters. Successful coaching practices mean we can look at the human as an individual entity with different requirements and goals that are constantly evolving. Each unique individual is at a different stage of physiological function and well-being. We just need to establish exactly where and what the logical path is from that stage.

Clinical practice allows us to understand many of the countless factors involved with the individual phenotype and its physiological potential; cellular growth rates, metabolic factors, cardiovascular and respiratory markers, and neural regulation to name but a few. The coach, more often than not, in the absence of a laboratory and clinical testing, is reliant on physiological feedback, observation, intelligent questioning, or trial and error to determine the most efficient path for the individual to move toward their desired goal.

We live in a world full of inherent risk factors that move us away from health and physiological and psychological well-being. We have the stress of modern life in both chronic and acute doses. We have obesity and physical inactivity exacerbated by the quality and quantity of energetic fuel. We have a plethora of diseased states and immune-compromising illnesses. All of these are part of the ever-changing hormonal landscape we live in. We must adapt our approaches to the individuals we deal with and provide environments that create healthy relationships both psychologically and physically with nutrition, training, and lifestyle.

THE BODY IS SMART

When considering energetic systems, remember the body is smart. It favors what we are good at and has pathways that are more efficient and appropriate for the task. In humans, some of the most important ones are the insulin and glucagon pathways. Our dependence on large amounts of carbohydrates as a fuel source means we are inefficient at smoothly transitioning between different energy substrates and using the inverse pathways offered to us by insulin and glucagon.

People who have indulged in carb-free or low-carb approaches will know what I mean that blunt period in which you are tired, lacking in fuel, and perhaps irritable, all to get you into a state you know is not manageable long term. We will discuss these more in chapter 12, as well as why we must use all the tools the body has and never hold sway in any one "camp" if we are to accomplish any level of flexibility in our approach to food. These two positions are commonly referred to as someone being either "carb-adapted" or "fat-adapted."

By continuing to eat in a particular regimented way, the dominant systems will adapt, and then possibly become overworked or overwhelmed; thus, over time, diminishing returns will be seen and ultimately, non-compliance will occur until the next dietary "system" is undoubtedly embarked upon. The problem we have is that these demands are often tainted by the day-to-day demands imposed on the body. These, in most cases, are impossible to avoid as much of what we do in day-to-day life, by nature, is imbalanced. Most of what we see in nutritional programming is designed for the "average" person; therefore, it negatively influences those that do not fit these average needs at that particular time.

We see other systems popularized and promoted by those who physiologically fit that method. Those who are already, or have always, maintained a relatively low level of body fat will be quick to promote nutritional systems that for the obese, or formerly obese, have minimal returns at that particular time. Yes, they may be sustainable systems, but they detract from the physiological and psychological needs of the client and their goals.

One of the reasons I never publish my diet is that it will be held in the belief, for the majority, that it is that diet that got me where I am today and not the one based on my current needs and demands. It evolved from something different. One of the things you will learn throughout this book is where to start and how to evolve these methods.

INDIVIDUAL CLIENT MANAGEMENT AND ASSESSMENT

From the initial contact with a client, it is critical that the process of gathering information pertaining to their requirements has begun. You can gather valuable information that will serve to ensure both client compliance and a successful outcome to the process and time spent.

How we would serve to gather this information is never-ending. Our senses become a tool; by observing, listening, and communicating, we collect new data. Noting the potentially compromised circulation upon shaking your client's hand can direct a line of questioning and reveal subtle clues that alone are small and may seem insignificant, but cumulatively can direct our efforts better.

Symptoms of poor circulation such as cold and numb hands or feet, hair loss in the legs or feet, and pale and cracked skin can all lead us to potentially damaged blood vessels and circulation. Clients who smoke, have high cholesterol, and/or have high blood pressure are all at risk. Diabetes, or the onset of diabetes coming about through uncontrolled and elevated blood glucose, can also damage blood vessels and thus circulation.

Every human being displays a series of characteristics both physiological and psychological. The process of assessment alongside both long- and short-term observation permits us to increase both the rate and frequency of success as coaches inordinately.

Within the world of coaching, the access and facility to undertake complex scientific testing is rare, so we rely heavily on what we observe in front of us and how, through experience, correct lines of questioning, and the understanding of both the science and literature on the topic, we can make better decisions.

Noting the subtle nuances between one physique and the next and responses to different stimuli means the actual "study group" we will deal with as coaches over the years will surpass any structured study. This however relies heavily on a coach who is attentive and not prejudicial in conclusions. Because a large part of a conclusion is often brought about by beliefs and theories, as opposed to science, coaches will bend the narrative using their knowledge and experience to support their beliefs at that particular time. It is critical therefore to keep an open mind and maintain a neutral, yet educated, approach. Opinions do exist and always will exist it is important to cultivate an educated opinion that can be swayed based upon new evidence.

In 2005, Hubal et al.[28] displayed the disparity in the physical development of humans. After studying 500 young, untrained, and healthy males through 12 weeks of progressive strength training, he found average strength levels went up by 54% and muscle mass went up by 19%. Probably the data most worthy of note was the variability with 0–250% for strength and -1–59% for muscle mass.[28]

The variety in stimulus versus outcome is huge; therefore, narrowing down what we can do with the tools we have at our disposal is critical to success.

GRASPING THE BASIC PSYCHOLOGY BEHIND FOOD CHOICES

Pay attention to hunger and how it affects your behavior. Consider times in which a food has been presented very well (even in a marketing sense) and it initiates a feeling of hunger or thirst that did not exist before. Let me present to you a picture of your favorite food right now. Look at it and acknowledge your feelings. If you are hungry, are your feelings different? If you have been restricting that food, are your feelings different? If someone has told you cannot have that food, are your feelings different?

The feelings are different, right? Our level of satiety will dictate a large portion of this, as well as the short-term pleasure that many seek from food the areas of the brain that lights up when people take pleasure from something. Addiction, as it is often defined in the case of food, is behavioral. The chemical properties of food are different than those of drugs and chemical variants, therefore rendering the "addiction" term not entirely factual.

Now imagine someone overweight who has even a small degree of metabolic dysfunction (which occurs prior to metabolic disease). This level of dysfunction can often be correlated alongside the level of obesity. Only in the case of metabolically benign obesity might this be different.

Those with these issues will more than likely have issues with the satiety hormones leptin, and ghrelin, alongside other metabolic hormones, such as insulin and glucagon. The satiety hormones signify starvation and send a signal to your brain to say, "Eat."

Someone with slight metabolic dysfunction is tantamount to having a mobile phone that you are starting to lose reception on. The more damage you do is equivalent to moving further and further from the cell tower. The communication becomes dull until it is practically nonexistent. People are not always hungry; they are merely getting a bad signal.

Now let me put this into context: someone shows a picture like the above and says, "You too can eat this and get lean, provided you stay within your calorie guidelines." Correct, but there is a small problem there. Psychology plays a large role, as does behavior, in what we eat. Now give someone who is overweight because of these metabolic dysfunctions a packet of biscuits when they are either hungry or in need of a pick-me-up and tell them they can only eat one. They may only eat one, but that false hunger signal that relies only on willpower to override it remains. In the majority of cases, it may over time become too overwhelming for many. Now you can possibly see why chronically low-calorie diets fail.

Those of you who are lean and have gone on a little food bender then struggle to get off it. Well, imagine that signal and the harsh reminders given to you by society every reflection you see and the numerous other factors that emphasize you are in a physical place you do not want to be.

The journey appears long and hard at this stage; for many, it is one they have consistently failed at and therefore it feels ominous and perhaps particularly with those that have never tried before unobtainable. This creates unhappiness and the cycle begins yet again. To offset the feeling, many reach for food or something else that may light up that same area of the brain: things influenced by culture, lifestyle, associations, and other cognitive factors. Food, if labeled as a reward, will create temporal happiness if you are unhappy. Food labeled as reward therefore creates pleasure.

If, as a coach, you are already lean and have good metabolic function, a level of empathy must be displayed alongside an understanding behind the psychological factors. For many people, we are aiming to get them to a place in which satiety signals are under better control. The psychology has been improved and perhaps associations detached and replaced with better relations with food. There are metabolic signals and simple things like past behavior that mean eating a scoop of ice cream as opposed the tub, a slice instead of the whole pizza, that need to be regulated.

Food is not addictive; there is nothing at all to clinically support this speculation. Food, and the way people perceive food, is a large part of the issue and it is a pleasurable pursuit. Maintain something that permits pleasure but also lends itself to better future practices and behavior. Make note of foods that may trigger irregular or past behaviors foods that may be associated with larger quantities of consumption or those related to events or situations: cinema trips, Friday nights, etc. Break habits, not willpower.

Flexibility within someone's diet is the dream we are striving for with our clients, but there is more to it than just telling the majority of people simply to count their macros and calories.

When you are physically happy, you look at the picture differently than when you are overweight. Those who have hands-on experience know this and understand this is behavior and psychology.

CHAPTER 4: PHYSIOLOGICAL CONSIDERATIONS

GENOTYPE, PHENOTYPE, AND SOMATOTYPE

An organism's genotype defines its fundamental hereditary information that which has been passed down from its parents or descendants, and that which is only really influenced in its expression. Its phenotype, however, is determined by factors such as its environment, morphology, development, and behavior. Consider the following as a way to view phenotype: Genotype + Environment + Interactions between Genotype and Environment = Phenotype. These are factored in over its existence and, as a result, are much more pliable by nature.

"Age is a period in which phenotype has had a smaller or greater length of time in which to influence the physiological and psychological well-being of someone. These influences could either be a positive or indeed negative manifestation.

At the stage of intervention and therefore apparent improvement of the phenotype, a coach must assess the degree, damage, or dysfunction that may have historically occurred. The older, therefore, someone is, the more damage could potentially have been done.

Age and degeneration is a linear relationship. We do however play a large role in the degree of that progressive degeneration."
~Phil Learney

The somatotype is seen largely as the outcome of interaction between both the genotype and phenotype. Several models have considered somatotypes. The one of most note is that of Sheldon and his now largely discredited model of constitutional psychology. His belief was that someone's body shape would determine and influence intellect, morality, and future successes. Despite the flaws in his study, it does provide us with valuable information about physiology and some noted differentials alongside physiological patterns that can influence our decision-making processes.[29]

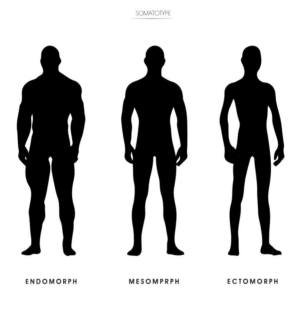

SOMATOTYPE

ENDOMORPH   MESOMPRPH   ECTOMORPH

Figure 3 Somatotypes.

Genotype appears to present us with three overlapping somatotypes.[30] The models overlap and a person is never of one distinct type; for most, their body is continually evolving in subtle fluxes, typically between two types. Somatypes help us by signifying physiological characteristics that could occur through genetic factors or those that, through phenotype, have been expressed differently or altered. For example, the wide shoulders and square jawline of the mesomorph indicates a higher level of both GH and free testosterone on a genetic level.

Although we cannot take this with clinical precision, it permits us the consideration of the phenotype right through to possibly childhood or into the early teen years and how influential our nutritional and training selection could potentially be. The genotype paints a better picture of the individual's physiological makeup and shows how dietary and environmental history may have influenced it.

We all note differences in physiques and the distinctions are perhaps clearer in their definitions. Genotype would have had less time in which interactions, including dietary and the psychological influence in dietary choices, can take hold. A snapshot of how someone was as a teenager may give us a better indication of what their genetic requirements may be.

To comprehend all influencing factors on human morphology would be impossible. However, things such as peer influence and social trends in both body image and dieting must not be disregarded. For example, those in their thirties or forties, particularly females, would have developed both physiological changes and psychological influences brought about by the low-fat and concurrently low-calorie dieting of that era. Men were not exposed heavily to aesthetic "expectancies" until probably the mid to late 1980s, so dietary culture had not yet taken hold.

Chronic low-calorie and low-fat dieting saw an increase or respective decrease in many endocrine markers, referred to clinically as neuroendocrine-immune dysfunction, and often resulted in prescriptive drug intervention when a marker was considered irregular. Poor testing methods (many of which still exist today), poor constructed clinical markers, and the lack of dietary consideration all share some degree of blame. A single marker above clinical guidelines would mean prescriptive drug intervention, whereas one marker below would be considered acceptable.

The influence of the media and peers on body image and the diet culture cannot be disregarded. One study found that over 50% of all 9–10 year old girls felt better about themselves when on a diet.[31] This somewhat disturbing statistic exemplifies the responsibility we have as figures of authority and influencers in dietary practices. We, alongside the people we influence, may ultimately be chasing a media- and society-driven ideal that may never be achieved. What is tantamount to our success as coaches is our ability to improve the perception these people have over their own bodies. Alongside a better, more sustainable, and healthier relationship with food, we encounter the favorable by-product of an improved body composition and health.

Look at the client's dietary history and note the chronological order of changes in both physiology and their perception of foods and foodstuffs. Look at current and historical trends in diets and using the upcoming notes on both caloric and macronutrient influences construct a strategic plan to rectify and positively affect the individual's rules pertaining to food and the acute and chronic changes that may have occurred physically and mentally.

Assess your own or your client's relationship with food. Is there a perception behind what is bad or what is good? Is there an agenda that serves to debase a food or food group unnecessarily? Is someone eradicating, cleansing, or fasting under the guise it is "good" for them, when they just want to lose weight but are not sure what to do about it? Educating these people and restoring balance to how they approach and perceive food is as much of a support to success as restoring someone's ability to self-regulate their intake of energy versus their energy requirements.

Despite Sheldon's model being discredited on a psychological level, it lends itself to noting a physiological difference in people's constitution and potential correlations with their macronutrient intake and requirements. It is not a "set" position someone remains in and in the fields of compositional change, it can often be used as a label to excuse an inability to lose fat, build muscle, etc. It must be understood that somatotype as aforementioned is indeed the interaction between genotype and phenotype, the latter of which we can influence enormously.

For example, a classically labeled ectomorph or "hard gainer" with a sound nutritional approach and training regimen may look, in later life, very different from their original or perceived somatotype. Studies have corroborated that ectomorphs do have a deficit in FFM and total body mass (TBM); the development over years in lean mass will influence the previous equation due to phenotype. There will always be traits present that could easily slide back into goal-compromising issues; however, if done steadily and with small steps, these are often sustainable changes.[32]

Any indication toward a particular somatotype may lead us to a different strategy simply by default and the suggestion that certain hormones may potentially dominate at the time of immediate assessment. In the absence of blood work or clinical assessment, it gives us another non-clinical tool to assess and correlate with the influence of phenotype: its relation to dietary and lifestyle history, current physiological status, and even its comparison to genotype. Those displaying an inclination toward an endomorph type would most certainly show a dietary history indicative of that phenotype. The key will be to note those of greatest negative influence and alter the trend.

People will genetically display differentials in their storage of energy in either fat or protein compartments. This again will have a reflective hormonal influence that undoubtedly correlates in some way.

How Relevant is This?

The influence of the environment, particularly dietary environment, largely influences physiological makeup. People, after all, are not born clinically obese. They may have either an increased or a decreased tendency to store fuel in fat compartments or perhaps have hormonal fluxes that mean lean tissue is harder to sustain or increase. However, like the variability in nutritional practices, these variables, if worked with correctly, can positively alter the physique of anyone.

Many aspects of the human physique are heritable yet environmentally modifiable and display a degree of biological plasticity. We are therefore constantly dealing with individuals at a transient and constantly evolving phase in their physiological development. They are in a stage we are attempting to influence the outcome of through sound nutritional advice and specific stimuli.

In striving to do this, we are trying to identify both the genotype and phenotype that has been evident throughout the individual's life span. Possibly the most influential and traceable therein is their nutritional history and their uninfluenced genetic "blueprint." Their past dietary forays low-carb, low-fat, and low-calorie diets and their various versions along the way should all be considered. The human phenotype is largely influenced by hormonal activity and hormonal activity is largely influenced by dietary habits. We will discuss the influence these dietary practices would have over phenotype later in the book.

Without an array of complex and often unavailable testing, are we in a position to visually assess what is in front of us and have an indirect insight into better programming choices? We are certainly in a position to ascertain the current status of an individual in a more comprehensive fashion through careful observation than through a few simple mathematical or generic prescriptions. In some cases, coaches will even replicate what worked personally for them across their clientele, as it becomes biased in its efficacy.

Our natural physiological makeup means that ratios of hormones will be unique and an integral part of our individual metabolic structure. Throughout the years, these will have adapted to and accommodated the stimuli we have given them or our environment has imposed upon them. Just like someone who opts for a high-pressure job will lend themselves to a higher level of catecholamines (stress hormones), the chronic nature of this environmental factor will influence the way in which the body metabolizes fuel and maintains its homeostatic control.

Those with a naturally high level of thyroid hormones will metabolize energy more efficiently. However, if under- or overstimulated for long enough, the body will adapt in an economical and efficient way. Irrespective of the natural physiological state, the phenotype will lead to a change: a change that is reflective of their current transient and morphological stage or somatotype.

It is our job to note these changes to the best of our abilities and make, what will be many, time-educated assumptions. These will mean that the inevitable process of trial and error becomes quantifiably shorter. We take what we can conclude and put it alongside that which we cannot and come up with a plan of best practices based upon it. We do not have the conclusive answer; however, we do have answers that serve a better outcome.

We have come very far from the days of simply counting calories or the caloric quality of food. Using the fundamental basis of thermodynamics considering energy in versus energy out as our sole model for compositional change would be short sighted. This is inevitably, however, the sum of the part we must work everything around, but it is not by any means the single factor.

We must look to macronutrients and the manipulation of them to work with the individual's current energy and substrate requirements. Acknowledging the current physiological and metabolic state of the individual will allow us to transiently move them to a state that is both manageable and sustainable considering their current physical and personal circumstances.

For example, an individual with a lower FFM would obviously spend more time in a caloric surplus to build and develop an increase in lean body mass (LBM). If considered alongside the genotype and phenotype, this implies a higher level of potential stress hormones, which would make the task of increasing LBM all the more difficult. A somatotype labeling of an ectomorph, in this case, only tells us where our challenges may fundamentally lie, but not the rationale behind why something cannot be done.

It is a matter of you, the coach, and the client overcoming the issue of a digestive system possibly influenced by the level of catecholamines alongside an inherent inability to consume adequate calories to potentiate an increase in LBM. I classify these people as "easy losers" as opposed to "hard gainers." In the battle of homeostasis, they spend more time in a catabolic or degenerative status than an anabolic or regenerative status. Often the focus lies with trying to gain as opposed to the much easier task of preventing loss.

We will focus on the nutritional implications later and how ever-changing phenotypes and genetic expression can alter our choices.

Chapter 5: Morphological Considerations

Morphology

The genetic makeup of people tells us males will be determined genetically by the XY chromosome and females by the XX chromosome. By this definition, the only influencing factor (as we cannot currently alter genetics) would be entirely hormonal. The biological sex of an individual will be determined by genitalia, the internal reproductive systems, the aforementioned chromosomes, hormonal levels, and the secondary sex characteristics such as breast tissue, hirsutism, and body fat distribution. We need to pay attention to what can be influenced and what cannot.

Genetics

When considering the genetic variability between individuals, we are looking at what is known as genetic polymorphisms.[33] These can be genetic variations or variability in DNA sequencing or chromosomes.

Polymorphisms have been primarily studied in relation to diseases and incidences in various human populations. It has been hypothesized that many dietary issues, such as lactose and carb intolerance may be associated with gene and nucleotide differentials. Let's consider lactose. In most mammals, including humans, the lactase enzyme responsible for the digestion of lactose in milk declines following the weaning phase; therefore, consumption of it beyond this point would lead to a food-based reaction that is not favorable.[34] However, the production of lactase into adulthood (termed "lactase persistence") is common in many humans. This is seen as a genetically inherited trait and is seen due to cis-acting polymorphism of lactase gene expression regulation.[35]

The relevance to such issues is most certainly of interest, but the inclusion or occlusion of things such as lactose from an individual's diet would simply be ascertained from their reaction post ingestion. We will not use an assumptive guess or removal simply because it might be a problem. Also, remember that the enzyme may simply be in a state where demand outweighs supply. Throughout life, the average adult may have ingested many foods because of dietary fads, their generational beliefs, or their culture in excessive quantities and overwhelmed the relevant production, supply, and demand chains of enzymes.

This does not mean all-out occlusion, but simply short-term lowering of, or omitting, the demand gives the supply chain chance to catch up. In the case of insulin, a temporary lowering of carbs and blood glucose may be appropriate, but long term, it would become counterproductive, as this will not only affect production, but also compromise the systems reliant on the functional macronutrient. It is a simple matter of better management of production, supply, and demand.

Research into genetics has shown us a correlation between the level of obesity and the production of salivary amylase, the enzyme responsible for the breakdown of starch within the digestive sequence.[36] A change in the number of genes is classed as copy number variations (CNVs) and this shows the subtle differences between individuals. When studying CNVs, we find the gene that makes amylase is AMY1 and can have up to 16 copies. The more of these copies, the more efficient you are at breaking down carbs in the digestive process. Data show variances in the genetic production of amylase and the association with high starch diets.[37–40]

There is not only genetic variation between individuals, but also in phenotypic variation. To look to genetic variables alone, without considering phenotype, would trick us into perhaps believing that it can be seen as the sole cause of any physiological issue. Someone simply overeating beyond their individual requirements cannot ever have their issues be entirely attributed to a genetic problem. Observations have certainly concluded that there are individuals who are more resistant to weight loss due to genetic influence. Reactiveness to chronic hyper- and hypocaloric diets appear to be influenced by genetic factors that we have yet to understand.[41]

Once again, I want to reiterate that there can be no single plan based upon a single parameter, percentage, or mathematical equation. Heredity, ethnicity, regional culture, dietary tradition, and the aforementioned factors must be considered when programming. An understanding of the regional cultures would most certainly play a part in the education of a good coach.

HOMEOBOX GENES

Homeobox genes (Gpc4, Tbx15, and, in particular, HoxA5) have an important role in the tissue patterning of humans during development. Evidence suggests that these contribute to the phenotypic characteristics of peripheral fat deposition and will play a role in the upper-lower (dorsal-ventral) and anterior-posterior patterning.[42–46]

Gene expression and heritability also contribute to distribution and locality of fat. It appears we can only influence this by altering the genetic expression brought about by diet and diet-induced obesity, insulin resistance, and overall adiposity. Improve these, and the gene expression appears to lend itself to more favorable outcomes. We cannot alter genes, but we can perhaps influence overall expression in a less complicated fashion than positive dietary intervention.[47]

In the absence of genetic testing, we can use the location of body fat and observation of secondary sex characteristics as a way to along with genotype, phenotype, and somatotype loosely determine current hormonal and physiological status to develop a better solution. There are, however, a few examples when the level of obesity does not correlate with the incidence of metabolic syndrome. In these examples, there is no apparent adverse metabolic profile–this is known as metabolically benign obesity. The odds, however, weigh in our favor that those with any significant level of obesity will more than likely display the characteristics of someone with metabolic syndrome.

METABOLIC SYNDROME

Metabolic syndrome is the term used for a series of metabolic dysfunctions that occur when the management of energy in both its direct usage and storage is compromised. It is most commonly seen to occur alongside pre-diabetes and obesity.[48]

The condition leads to deterioration in the management of insulin by the pancreas and a concurrent increase in the risk of cardiovascular disease. Numerous biomarkers occur in the presence of metabolic syndrome. These could include an elevation in blood pressure, decreased fasting serum high-density lipoprotein (HDL) cholesterol, elevated fasting serum triglyceride level, impaired fasting glucose, insulin resistance, or pre-diabetes. These all are precursors to medically diagnosed and metabolically diseased states.

Associations have also been shown between metabolic syndrome and polycystic ovary syndrome (PCOS) and an increase in the presence of uric acid within the blood, decrease in total testosterone, and erectile dysfunction.[49]

In noting the accumulation of such signs and symptoms, it would lead the more analytical of us down a more complex route to find a solution to each issue. The collection of issues appears to resonate largely from poor dietary habits and a single point, so rectification of such dysfunctions appears largely to revolve around better and more sustainable dietary habits.

This reversal of habitually poor dietary habits in many cases will affect, cumulatively and positively, nearly all issues mentioned. The complication simply lies in good nutritional planning and structure. Medical and pharmacological science may overlay short-term intervention for some symptoms, but do not detract from the power of good nutritional practices.

LOCATION OF BODY FAT

Studies have shown that the location of body fat can be used to outline three fundamental body types: gynoid (pear-shaped), intermediate, and android (apple-shaped), all of which will be determined at the genetic level by skeletal structure and the aforementioned gene-by-sex locality of fat distribution.[50]

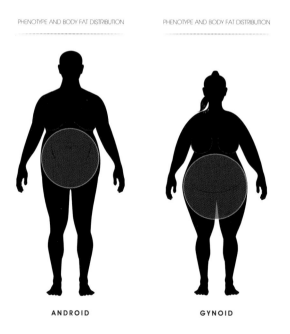

Figure 4 Gynoid and android body classifications alongside body fat distribution.

Gynoid fat distribution (more clinically termed "gluteofemoral fat") is evidenced by a lower-body subcutaneous fat pattern. Android fat distribution is evidenced by an intra-abdominally localized fat pattern (apple-shaped) and, in most cases, is visceral fat. It should be noted that fat stored in the abdominal area has a greater effect on cardiovascular health compared to fat stored in the hip and thigh region.

Visceral fat in this particular phenotype would indicate a higher likelihood of insulin resistance, higher total cholesterol, higher low-density lipoprotein (LDL) (bad) cholesterol, and lower HDL (good) cholesterol. The only scenario in which this would not be the case would be if someone had the aforementioned metabolically benign obesity. This would suggest that, despite the level of obesity, it is largely subcutaneous fat and, therefore, will not be accompanied by insulin resistance and early stages of arteriosclerosis.[51]

Visceral fat responds very well to diet and exercise, and subcutaneous fat poses very little risk to health. Studies have shown that removal of subcutaneous fat shows no difference in health markers than you would see from a reduction in visceral deposits.[52]

This does not detract from the fact that, from the aesthetic perspective, most people are still more concerned about the visual reduction in subcutaneous fat as opposed to the health benefits seen through visceral fat reduction. The favorable fact is that in lowering someone's overall body fat, there is the welcome by-product that visceral fat will decrease as well, followed thereafter by subcutaneous fat levels.

Distribution of body fat appears to have a strong heritable component and is largely genetically and hormonally regulated.[53] Studies analyzing the relationship between body build and hormone levels have shown us that estradiol levels were understandably highest in gynandromorphic men and lowest in mesomorphic men.[54]

Dehydroepiandrosterone sulfate (DHEA-S), testosterone levels, and hirsutism (excessive hair growth) have been shown to be higher in those displaying centralized fat distribution, as opposed to those with lower-body fat distribution. Mesomorphic body types are likely to have higher levels of these, but lower levels of estrogen.[55, 56] Estrogen will be higher in those displaying gynoid body fat distribution (and potentially female sex characteristics in males), gynecomastia (development of breast tissue), and the thinning of connective tissue surrounding the reproductive organs, potentially resulting in visual signs of cellulite.

Estrogen appears to play a significant role in the accumulation of lower-body fat in females. The inclination that we must lower estrogen is often misconstrued when, in fact, the dynamic ratio between testosterone and estrogen simply needs to be improved. The support, in many cases, is that testosterone lends itself to a better ratio and better distribution of body fat. In summary, locality of body fat will influence certain hormonal markers. This cannot obviously be clinically accurate without adequate testing, but we can make better conclusions based upon a higher likelihood.

Often, clinical issues surround these hormone levels due to poor lab testing in both males and females. Elevation or deficiency is often caused by a change in the dynamic ratio, increased sensitivity to androgens or estrogens, or, in some cases, a high level of aromatization (the conversion of androgens to estrogens). Aromatase activity has been shown to increase in response to obesity, insulin, and elevation in the follicle-stimulating hormone (FSH), luteinizing hormone (LH), and placental chorionic hormone human chorionic gonadotropin (hCG). The testing undertaken often fails to look at the bigger picture.

Further into the text, we will consider the implications brought about by the rate or incremental path of weight and/or fat loss. Those with short-term imposed deadlines will have the need to simply camp in the hypocaloric states necessary for weight loss. As this lends itself to poor support of the hypothalamic–pituitary–adrenal (HTPA) axis, it becomes, over time, compromised through the adaptation of metabolic processes leading to weight loss, particularly fat loss slowing. Long term, it can also support metabolic dysfunction and its irregular behavioral patterns.

This hormonal influence negatively affects the support of testosterone as the rate and time in a hypocaloric state is simply too harsh and extreme. This type of aggressive dieting can also influence receptor sites that then influence proportional fat distribution. Only in the case of pharmacological intervention can such steep incremental fat loss regimens be effective in overall fat loss. Even then, the pharmacological support can cause further issues.

Dieting for longer and steadier periods of times supports current receptor makeup, the hormonal axis, sustainability, and overall dietary compliance. The sucker punch for many is that it requires an amount of patience that many people are not prepared to give they want a small prize now, as opposed to a big prize later. [57]

The more obese people become, the more impatient they often are to change com-positionally. Many happily forego the "big prize" later for the "small prize" now. Being a good coach means being able to empathize and be honest about the length of the journey they are about to embark upon honesty and integrity play as much of a role as knowledge. These people have been sold, quite literally in many cases, "the dream" too many times.

Ask them, "If I was to sit down with you a year from now and you were to be largely content with your body, and in addition to this, you were able to maintain that physique with both a good family and social life, would this make you happy? If the journey that you had just undertaken had brought along with it far more pleasurable and positive experiences than just pain, would you take it?"

Given that almost all sexual differentiation outside of genetics is a result of hormonal fluctuations, we can use this as largely a sliding scale. This resonates from the genetic start point from which someone began and, from that point, how hormonal alterations may have influenced their developmental characteristics. We can only attempt to reset someone's base point: the enhancement of it beyond speculative pharmaceutical intervention is impossible.

This simple fact debunks the notion that lifting weights or any type of positive nutritional intervention, as a single entity, can masculinize females. It can only serve to capitalize on what is already genetically set or available. The case in which masculinization could occur is when there is an impact on aromatization brought about by a disruption in the balance of androgens and estrogen something training is simply incapable of.

In PCOS, the ovaries lose the dynamic balance of hormones, thus producing a higher level of androgens. Insulin, alongside LH, acts on the ovaries, stimulating them to produce more testosterone. These high levels of insulin, LH, and testosterone interfere with the follicle development in the ovaries, meaning many become underdeveloped. This mainly affects ovulation and fertility, but excess of testosterone can lead to levels of masculinization. This can be associated with, but certainly not directly linked to, an individual's level and distribution of subcutaneous body fat.

PCOS is a cascade effect from many hormones and has no singular cause; however, most notably, insulin and the development of insulin resistance appear to have a large part to play in the condition. For many, positive compositional and dietary changes are adequate enough to reverse the dysfunction brought about by insulin resistance. The other such incidence of masculinization and feminization is when exogenous androgens are used, thus chemically altering the HTPA axis.

CHAPTER 6: HOMEOSTASIS AND ALLOSTASIS

HOMEOSTASIS AND ALLOSTASIS

We are all in a constant state of stimulation with environmental, physical, and nutritional stimuli of most concern to us. The body adapts to this stimuli through a series of homeostatic and allostatic controls. These controls maintain a dynamic balance between the autonomic branches: the sympathetic, which supports the fight-or-flight response, and parasympathetic, which supports the rest-and-digest response. Modern life often disrupts this homeostatic control.

There are several theories behind homeostasis and its regulatory mechanisms. We will not get into the debatable intricacies and differentials between homeostasis and allostasis, but consider them as collective terms used for the regulation of systems and internal stability within the body. Homeostasis literally means, "standing at about the same level," whereas allostasis means, "remaining stable by being variable": one of which appears uniform in its role, whereas the other is highly dynamic. We must adapt on both levels, so the need to differentiate between them is unnecessary for the sake of our discussion. We need to see it largely as a transparent occurrence.

Allostatic control will see changes in physiology and psychology in the midst of altering variables. Stress, activity level, poor dietary habits, behavior, overall composition, and, of course, aging. To maintain life, there will be alterations in the HTPA axis, the autonomic nervous system, cytokines, and other systems throughout this time.[58–62]

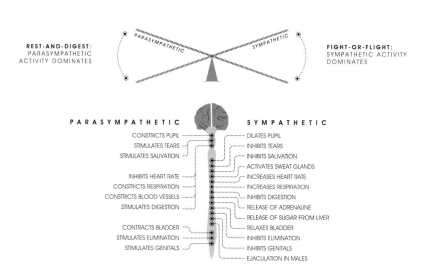

HOMEOSTASIS IS A DYNAMIC BALANCE BETWEEN THE AUTONOMIC BRANCHES

REST-AND-DIGEST:
PARASYMPATHETIC
ACTIVITY DOMINATES

FIGHT-OR-FLIGHT:
SYMPATHETIC ACTIVITY
DOMINATES

PARASYMPATHETIC

- CONSTRICTS PUPIL
- STIMULATES TEARS
- STIMULATES SALIVATION
- INHIBITS HEART RATE
- CONSTRICTS RESPIRATION
- CONSTRICTS BLOOD VESSELS
- STIMULATES DIGESTION
- CONTRACTS BLADDER
- STIMULATES ELIMINATION
- STIMULATES GENITALS

SYMPATHETIC

- DILATES PUPIL
- INHIBITS TEARS
- INHIBITS SALIVATION
- ACTIVATES SWEAT GLANDS
- INCREASES HEART RATE
- INCREASES RESPIRATION
- INHIBITS DIGESTION
- RELEASE OF ADRENALINE
- RELEASE OF SUGAR FROM LIVER
- RELAXES BLADDER
- INHIBITS ELIMINATION
- INHIBITS GENITALS
- EJACULATION IN MALES

Figure 5 Impact of the fight-or-flight response on the HTPA axis. Illustration of response, from the hypothalamus to neural activity.

Sterling proposed six interrelated principles that underlie allostasis:
- Organisms are designed to be efficient.
- Efficiency requires reciprocal trade-offs.
- Efficiency also requires being able to predict future needs.
- Such prediction requires each sensor to adapt to the expected range of input.
- Prediction also demands that each effector adapts its output to the expected range of demand.
- Predictive regulation depends on behavior while neural mechanisms also adapt.[63]

If we consider the principles Sterling proposes, we can grasp that there is a period of adaptation to anything. Undoubtedly, the organism becomes efficient over this period. To burn or metabolize fuel efficiently, we must be inefficient in the process, but efficient in the mechanisms that drive it. For example, we want to be efficient in the passage of foodstuffs through digestive processes. Once in the body, however, we want inefficiency to use nutrients.

THE HTPA AXIS

The HTPA axis is the collective feedback loop and interaction between the three glands it is named after: the hypothalamus, pituitary, and adrenal glands. Together, they serve as the control mechanism of the body in response to stress, regulating the immune system, digestion, psychological state, and storage and expenditure of energy.

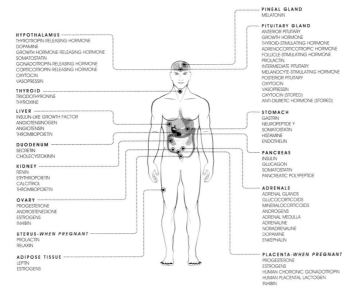

Figure 6 The endocrine system.

The hypothalamus is the central hub of this system and manages the body's autonomic responses. In a state of excitement, stressors signal the hypothalamus to release corticotropin-releasing hormone (CRH); in turn, this activates the pituitary. The pituitary gland, also known as the "master gland," then secretes a number of hormones particularly adrenocorticotropic hormone (ACTH) into the bloodstream, acting on the adrenal cortex and releasing cortisol into the bloodstream. Cortisol and ACTH are rhythmically secreted throughout the day and coordinated with the circadian rhythm, meaning both peak early morning and hit minimum late afternoon and evening.

We will talk about the specific hormones in chapter 13, but the pituitary gland can be split into the anterior and posterior portions.

HORMONAL RESPONSIBILITIES

THE ANTERIOR PITUITARY

ACTH	Stimulates glucocorticoid and androgen release
GH	Works in opposition to insulin and stimulates insulin-like growth factor-1 (IGF-1)
LH and FSH	Release sex steroids
Prolactin	Responsible for lactation and growth of the reproductive organs
Thyroid- stimulating hormone(TSH)	Stimulates the release of thyroxine (T4)

THE POSTERIOR PITUITARY

Anti-diuretic hormone (ADH)	Acts on the kidneys to prevent water excretion
Oxytocin	Assists the myoepithelial cells in contracting and releasing breast milk

THE HYPOTHALAMUS

Growth-hormone-releasing hormone (GHRH)	Increases the release of GH
Growth-hormone-inhibiting hormone (GHIH),	also known as somatostatin Decreases the release of GH and TSH
CRH	Increases the release of ACTH
Gonadotropin-releasing hormone (GnRH)	Increases LH and FSH
Thyrotropin-releasing hormone (TRH)	Increases TSH and prolactin
Prolactin-releasing factors (PRF)	Increases prolactin release
Dopamine (prolactin -inhibiting hormone)	Decreases prolactin

Once the pituitary gland has released ACTH, the adrenal glands come into play. These release and synthesize the hormones responsible for dealing with any kind of imposed stress. Elevation of cortisol and catecholamines such as adrenaline (epinephrine) and noradrenaline (norepinephrine) all result in the shutdown of the body's non-essential systems. Digestion and nutrient turnover are inhibited. Alongside this, heart rate increases, pupils dilate, breathing rate increases, sweat glands are activated, and blood vessels constrict. Glucose is released from the liver as fuel. All of this happens just to deal with an imposed threat.[64]

This is the sympathetic side of the nervous system working. In opposition to these reactions, the parasympathetic nervous system (PSNS) serves to counteract and re-establish homeostatic control.

Chapter 7: The Nervous System and Adrenals

We can subdivide the autonomic (involuntary) nervous system into two parts: the SNS and PSNS. We must also consider the enteric nervous system (ENS), which is the term often used for the actions of the digestive system. The SNS is responsible for the fight-or-flight response initiated under situations of threat. In response to this, the body primes itself to run or fight. The adrenal medulla, part of the adrenal gland, secretes catecholamines, particularly epinephrine (adrenaline), norepinephrine (noradrenaline), and dopamine. This is of concern to us due to the increase in heart rate, blood pressure, blood vessel constriction, and therefore the subsequent increase in both metabolism and lipolysis. Epinephrine is also the primary hormone that stimulates fat loss.[65]

In states of hypoglycemia, which are preempted by low blood sugar, the function of the brain will down-regulate. This not only results in an alteration in energy and mood, but long term can lead toward anxiousness, depression, and overall fatigue. When the HTPA axis recognizes low blood sugar, it releases epinephrine into the system, allowing blood glucose to rise. It also facilitates, alongside norepinephrine, the release of free fatty acids (FFAs) into plasma.[66]

This entire process may create a feeling much like anxiety, alterations in breathing, and nervousness. Some of you may have experienced this an hour or two after an intensive workout or in anticipation of a big event (or leg day). This is partly due to epinephrine being released to fuel the brain and the body getting ready to fight.

To create equilibrium and prevent the body from essentially burning out, the PSNS opposes the above by initiating a state of calm with its cholinergic nerves by releasing acetylcholine and reestablishing regular homeostatic function. Both are important when considering compositional change, as we live in a chronically overstimulated society. As you can see, the benefits of the nervous system to the trainee are enormous, but stress must be monitored and accounted for. Lifestyle, nutrition, and training alongside the personality characteristics of the individual must be considered.

The ENS governs the gastrointestinal system.[67] It coordinates interactions innervating the walls of the gastrointestinal tract, signaling the hormones and chemical messengers that largely influence food intake and satiety signals. The two catecholamines responsible for regulating lipolysis (fat breakdown) are epinephrine and norepinephrine, both of which act on alpha- and beta-adrenergic receptors.

Two major types of adrenoreceptors that influence fat metabolism are of interest to us. Alpha-2 adrenoreceptors have lower sympathetic innervation and inhibit lipolysis (fat breakdown), decrease blood flow through adipose tissue, and stimulate overall fat cell numbers. Beta-2 adrenoreceptors have greater sympathetic innervation and increase both blood flow and the level of lipolysis. The differing distribution of subcutaneous fat would lead us to think that, in areas that show higher levels of stored fat, there will also be a higher level of alpha-2 adrenoreceptors. Hence, despite fat loss being widely accepted as an evenly distributed occurrence, it is not.[68] These receptors would also partly explain an individual's predisposition to fuel storage in either lean or fat compartments.

This differential in body fat distribution comes with other issues when it includes lipolysis. Alpha-2 adrenoreceptors are more abundant in gluteofemoral, or lower-body, fat. Beta-receptors therefore are more abundant in intra-abdominal fat. Thus, when we consider "stubborn" areas lower back, abs, etc. there is an association with an increase in those areas to the number of alpha-2 receptors.

Compound this with the fact that males typically have more adrenal receptors intra-abdominally, whereas women display more around the hip and thigh (gluteofemoral) region and this would explain the phenomenon of female athletes who get very lean in the upper body but the hips and thighs remain far behind in progress. This would also suggest that indirect "spot reduction" is actually theoretically possible; much like "spot accumulation" appears indirectly possible. The fat patterning we discussed earlier and the gynoid and android shapes will show a higher amount of the anti-lipolytic alpha-receptors in the regions predisposed to higher fat levels.

To use fat from these stubborn areas it is often simply a matter of persistence. A female or even a male with this higher concentration of alpha-receptors in any area of adipocytes will see that both mobilization and utilization as fuel will be slower and perceived as stubborn. Incredibly lean areas with a higher concentration of beta-receptors will then and only then rely on the other compartments for fuel.

A longer duration of dieting is often the resolution to such an issue. The ratio of alpha- to beta-receptors in an adipocyte, as well as localized blood flow, will therefore be a large factor in the rate of fat loss in any particular cell.

In my experience, the concentration of localized and "stubborn" body fat appears to be at higher levels in those with a history of being overweight or obese because they have altered receptor makeup and concentration.

These areas all appear to be notably slower in response to fat loss and seem to respond better to much less aggressive strategies. It could be assumed that this is caused by a higher concentration of alpha-receptors. However, from my observations, the longer and more steadily nutrition is regulated, the more even the distribution becomes over time. As historical patterns typically stem from irregularity, for these people, the success often lies in achieving compliance and regulation.

We must also consider blood flow. Without adequate blood flow to fat cells, the hormones responsible for lipolysis cannot perform their actions. Fat may be mobilized from elsewhere but remain stagnant in stubborn areas. This is a compounded problem; a higher concentration of alpha-receptors means there is inhibited blood flow in the tissue. As vasoconstriction increases, it also bluntly inhibits lipolysis. Concentrations of beta cells have the opposing effect: increasing blood flow due to vasodilation and lipolysis. Without blood flow, the FFA cannot be moved away from the adipocyte to be used as fuel. Increasing blood flow to a specific area may hypothetically increase the rate of lipolysis in that area.

STIMULATING THE RECEPTORS

Now that we understand more about the receptors that influence fat metabolism, we can use that knowledge to our advantage. When we diet in any hypocaloric state, there is a drop in sympathetic activity by the nervous system, which results in a drop in both metabolic rate and lipolysis.

To stimulate this activity, we have the cyclical use of nutrients and calories that will offset this chronic slowing. We also have the potential to offset this slowing using stimulants or receptor antagonists such as caffeine and yohimbine, both of which will ask the adrenoreceptors to work beyond their homeostatic levels. However, due to the adaptation of such stimuli over time, the returns can diminish. Caffeine affects the SNS by inhibiting phosphodiesterase and preventing the breakdown of adenosine.[69] This blocks the adenosine, causing a rise in the other neurotransmitters and results in an increase in both epinephrine and norepinephrine.[70] Caffeine blocks the receptor from receiving adenosine. Adenosine is a neuromodulator that acts as both an activator and inhibitor and when it cannot do its job, the stimulatory effects of caffeine are enhanced. If you sleep well at night, the adenosine facilitates this through its ability to bind to receptors.

Because the adenosine molecules are blunted from attaching to receptors by the caffeine (caffeine is what we call an adenosine-receptor antagonist), once the caffeine clears, a large amount of non-cleared and dormant adenosine hits the receptors all at once. The ensuing tiredness means the average person will undoubtedly reach for another caffeine hit, yet again blocking the adenosine temporarily instead of letting it clear.

Long-term stimulation or blocking of receptors can result in the adrenals becoming fatigued. When the body is put under any chronic or intensely acute organic stress even that which stimulants would induce over time, this will cause a diminished hormonal response and potential physical dependence.[71]

Without moving into the intensive psychology behind this, most of what we encounter with levels of anxiety will be accompanied by decreased appetite.[72,73] Observationally, if we consider somatotypes of all the preceding traits, you may find higher frequency in ectomorphs and hypertensive subjects.[74]

These are what we term "vegetative" functions and their disruption can indicate levels of emotional stressors. Whenever these are observed, it is advisable to try to minimize the non-organic stressors, such as stimulants, from their nutrition.[75] It is worth noting that many dysfunctional eating patterns begin in times of heightened anxiety, stress, etc. Trying to ascertain dietary patterns that occur around these emotional disturbances may give us direction with our emotional or support mechanisms.

Griffin[75] noted the strong emotional significance of food and the feelings of security, comfort, and happiness that are often brought about by patterns solidified during infancy. It is suggested that these patterns may be a factor in some cases of obesity and, without doubt, in any degree of disordered eating.[75]

However, despite caffeine increasing resting energy expenditure (REE) and promoting both lipolysis and fatty acid oxidation, it must be noted that high body stores of carbohydrate and/or ingestion will minimize the rise in serum FFA levels

brought about by the consumption of caffeine. Therefore, if fat loss is a goal, caffeine is best used when carbohydrate levels are low and when the client is on a hypocaloric diet.[76—78]

Remember, when using anything that acts to stimulate receptors, we must always consider that these receptors will down-regulate, thus requiring more over time to do the same job. Over time, this puts excessive demands on the glands. Caffeine is a tool that can be used in periods of low energy and when carbohydrates are low. It will only notably affect fat loss in these conditions, so if the intent is to use it for its ergogenic properties, reserve the heightened use of it until you are already pretty lean.

UNDERSTANDING AGONISTS AND ANTAGONISTS

Agonists will bind to the receptors, creating a positive action, whereas an antagonist will bind and inhibit it. For fat loss, we need to stimulate specific receptors and, in turn, the SNS to mobilize fat for use as fuel.

Consider the example of beta-blockers. This class of drugs (receptor antagonists) inhibits the action of stress hormones or endogenous catecholamines through v asoconstriction (the narrowing of blood vessels) as opposed to dilation. These serve to dampen the fight-or-flight response and impact of adrenaline and noradrenaline.

When considering fat loss, we must be in a physiological state to use fat as energy. An acute rise in stress hormones alongside a lowered level of insulin will cause glucagon its opposing hormone to signal adipocytes to release their stores of fat to be used as fuel.

Without the initial mobilization of fatty acids, the body will continue to store fat while using other substrates, including its own tissue, as fuel. This is what we are trying to avoid and one of the reasons intensive exercise helps us not only preserve muscle mass but also mobilize fatty acids.

This relies on not only the release of catecholamines, glucagon, and various other hormones that will activate lipase the enzyme responsible for breaking down fat but also on increased blood flow. Anything that vasoconstricts will inhibit all of the actions acting upon the adipocytes, so these actions cannot occur.

Areas with both high concentrations of alpha-receptors and poor circulation will thus have trouble mobilizing and using fatty acids as fuel (hips on those with predominant gynoid distribution, the abdomen in those with android distribution). Encouraging not only a release in fatty acids but also a mobilization of them by an increase in blood flow would be beneficial in all cases.

In response to stress, the body releases epinephrine from the SNS. Adipose tissue and muscle tissue have a large amount of adrenergic receptors on their surface[79] that allow epinephrine to bind to them. Through the stimulation of several proteins and activation of the enzymes, there is a conversion of adenosine triphosphate (ATP) into cyclic adenosine monophosphate (cAMP), binding then to protein kinase A. Protein kinase A releases a subunit that phosphorylates hormone-sensitive lipase (HSL), allowing triglycerides to be broken down into both glycerol and fatty acids to be used as energy.

This breakdown of triglycerides and fatty acids is critical if fat loss is the goal. Increasing levels of obesity mute the impact epinephrine has on HSL; therefore, there is an increased demand for epinephrine to be able to break down and mobilize triglycerides.

In contrast, a metabolically trained individual is able to enhance the efficiency of the mobilization and breakdown. Aerobic exercise that creates a metabolic training effect cannot only enhance the mobilization and breakdown of fat, but the enhanced circulation can also help increase blood flow through the areas with lower sympathetic innervation and higher concentration of alpha-receptors.

Fat Storage Utilization, Mobilization, and Transport

During hypercaloric intake beyond requirements, adipocytes (fat cells) remove lipids from the bloodstream for storage (lipogenesis). In contrast, when an energy deficit is caused by a hypocaloric restriction or energy demand, the adipocytes release fatty acids for use as fuel (lipolysis). In the case of surplus energy, fat cells in a similar fashion to muscle go through a stage of hypertrophy (enlargement).

 Once at a critical level of mass, it is hypothesized that they proliferate and cause hyperplasia, which is an increase in the number of adipocytes.[80] Hyperplasia of adipocytes, much like in muscle tissue, has research behind it, but is deemed to only occur at certain stages of life or in extreme physiological circumstances.[81,82] Adipocytes are cells that store energy as fat. These are inclusive of the two types of fat: white adipose tissue and brown adipose tissue.

Understanding the current physiological position of an individual puts us in a much better position to construct a strategy for compositional change. We have adequate science and knowledge and, by using the right observations and lines of questioning, we are able to make educated initial decisions. Once the process begins, this is an ongoing assessment that will be adjusted by further evidential data and simple trial and error. We must always consider genotype and include what we know of both their past and present nutritional habits to form a strategy.

CHAPTER 8: THE NUTRITION

Ultimately, our goal is to establish a sustainable way for someone to make better nutritional choices that lead to improvements in both their physical and psychological well-being.

Empowering people to make sustainable nutritional choices requires giving them the tools they need to manage their food choices so they are compatible with both their lifestyle and their own evolving physiology. We must educate and empower people to deal with the enormous pressure society places on physical image and our own psychology.

By studying both habitual and learned behaviors, as well as considering what people may have experienced in their childhood, we can begin to look at not only the mathematical side of nutritional programming, but also the more complex issues surrounding adherence.

Certain foods from our childhoods have become linked to specific emotions and behaviors. Some foods may simply remind us of pleasurable times or events. Others may have been treated as rewards and ingrained as such. These associations and learned behaviors are part of operant (or instrumental) conditioning. These would have been reinforced not only by our parents and their previous learned behaviors, but also by anyone who has intervened in our nutritional habits throughout life, including coaches.[83]

There is never a single nutritional system to follow, but rather an ever-evolving series of phasic and systematic choices. Grasping the theory and science behind many of these pre-designed systems and their purposes permits us to adapt them according to individual and circumstantial requirements. The goal is to develop a broader understanding of influential factors and learn how we can alter a client's physiological status through both nutrition and behavior.

BUILDING A NUTRITIONAL STRATEGY

Now it is time to make some decisions. First, make sure you are clear on the goals whether your own or your client's. Next, you must determine how best to integrate the pursuit of those goals within that individual's lifestyle. From this, we can form an initial plan that can be adjusted, adapted, and amended as required.

There is never an intelligently designed system that completely fails simply one with flaws. Perhaps the scenario of missing a meal and an aversion to low blood glucose causes you to crave high-sugar foods. Perhaps miscalculating caloric intake and output creates chronic hunger. Perhaps there is metabolic signaling dysfunction.

These are the issues we must address and the flaws we must work out of the system. We should oppose imposing inherent sentiments, supporting the feelings of failure society creates, and the old adage that our only weakness is a lack of willpower. There is more to success than simply eating less, training more, and having a coach that spews motivational quotes.

Without getting into incredibly heavy science right now (which isn't really the onus of this text), the hormonal signaling that occurs with increased adiposity is, for the most part, a mess.

For many, losing body fat is hard. Pushed by goals to reach a "societal norm" and believing "restriction" is a preferred dietary modality, anything remotely normal or sustainable is often far from people's scope of view. Pushing them to own what they do now is not a promise of a magic pill or an outstanding short-term physical transformation: it becomes something that will empower them to take emotional and physical control of themselves, their life, and their results.

THE CATCH

If composition is a concern, overeating will always result in the need, at some stage, to undereat. Both over- and undereating have their relative and unavoidable trade-offs. Much like searching the internet for a better price because too much money was spent shopping last time, we often undereat to control or minimize the cost of overeating.

At this stage, consistently adhering to any plan, coupled with sporadic energetic input and output, will bring about changes for many people changes they have never before achieved. To lead the body beyond this stage is tantamount to a having a road under construction. Although roads may close temporarily or cause stopped traffic while under construction, when completed, they are resurfaced and work much more efficiently.

The body is composed of numerous systems that, at times, need stress alleviated from them. To say this would not become restrictive at times in the short term would be misleading and somewhat delusional. The short-term omittance of any type of food is done to "resurface the street," so to speak. The "roads" will all open again.

The long-term goal is to put the individual in a position where almost any road is efficient and passable. When considering that the average human rotates 20–30 varying foods, choosing different streets while the others are repaired is actually pretty easy. Couple that with the enormous adaptive capabilities of the human body, and we simply need a plan and an intelligent strategy that stems from their current physiological position.

MEAL FREQUENCY

When deciding on meal frequency, numerous overlapping factors must be considered. First, is what you choose indefinitely sustainable? This is a critical aspect of long-term nutrition plans and sadly is grossly overlooked by many when structuring eating plans. Remember that multiple meals can take longer to prepare and time must be available for increased meal frequency.

Many people aspiring to achieve physique improvements blindly continue to follow the bodybuilding norm of high-frequency feedings (six to eight meals a day). This has been somewhat perpetuated by the concept that it will notably influence fat loss metabolism or metabolic rate. However, in many cases, it may actually slow this process, so it must be considered carefully.

There is no substantial evidence to support that an increase in meal frequency affects thermogenesis. Therefore, eating little and eating often does not positively influence weight loss. In some cases, it makes the consumption of calories in hypercaloric diets somewhat easier.[84–90] But for many, high meal frequency is unnecessary and unsustainable.

If composition is our primary goal, one of our main nutritional priorities in choosing meal frequency is to positively influence the body's amino acid pool. Ensuring the body has a readily available source of amino acids means our risk of long-term lean tissue loss (or even limiting lean tissue gains) is managed. It also supports recovery from intensive exercise and helps maintain our adaptive reserve.

During periods of hypocaloric dieting, it has been shown (under the assumption protein levels are adequate) that meal frequency can potentially help preserve lean mass in trained populations. This is supported by the fact that protein breakdown (or oxidation) is increased and nitrogen loss is decreased in lower meal frequencies (three meals or less).[91,92]

Amino acids from whole food sources give us roughly five to eight hours before our bodies use our own physical stores of amino acids for repair or even fueling. Should the body be devoid of all other caloric- and energy-yielding substrates, it is a simpler process than the breakdown and use of stored fat. For anyone seeking optimal physical and, particularly, lean tissue, this development would lead you to question the classic three meal structure of Western society. Compound this with the fact most Western diets are devoid of adequate protein and tissue management could be a long-term complication to ongoing metabolic turnover rates.

A minimum of four feedings, containing a whole food protein source, per day would likely be more beneficial than the three feeding structure and more than adequate in most cases. Ideally, meal frequency should be evenly split over the waking hours in a 24-hour period. This supports not only lean tissue sparing, but also less hepatic stress due to the positive influence on insulin concentrations.[93,94]

WHEN DOES THIS CHANGE?

There are numerous physiological situations in which it would be suggested to increase or decrease meal frequency. However, these are never a suitable trade-off for a sustainable long-term pattern. It would not be detrimental to fluctuate between meal frequencies, but it would complicate the nutritional plan and would be unsustainable.

Carefully consider the meal frequency decision because, for many, it can make or break compliance. In many, the decreased hunger and appetite control brought about by increased frequency are largely beneficial for those susceptible to hypoglycemic bouts.[95–97]

An increase in meal frequency supports and benefits those with any level of insulin resistance or any form of diabetes. The literature supports that increased frequency of eating leads to better blood glucose control and numerous other cholesterol health markers.[98]

Therefore, those with any sign of metabolic syndrome may initially benefit from an increase in meal frequency because more stable blood glucose lends itself to controlling potential binge episodes brought about by unstable levels. This simultaneously decreases resistance and increases sensitivity to insulin.

Increased meal frequency also benefits bodybuilders aiming to increase mass as their main priority. Despite a lack of research, when considering muscular gain, the fact is that a caloric surplus must be achieved irrespective of anything else.[99] Consumption of more frequent meals will assist somewhat with turnover; increased meal frequency has been shown to support nitrogen loss and lipid oxidation and encourages the pancreas to produce a less acute amount of meal-induced insulin.

The more insulin stimulated, the more we stimulate the glucose transporter type four (GLUT-4) transporters that allow greater uptake of glucose into cells while minimizing acute hepatic stress. This overlaps and supports a sustained increase in potential workout volume critical in itself to lean mass gain. Also, despite needing significantly more research, the data related to sarcopenia and rate of protein synthesis seem to be in favor of higher frequency feedings. However, this does not necessarily correlate to changes in muscular levels.[100–102]

This is not to categorically say that more is better; but in some cases, increased meal frequency may lead to better compliance due to a more stable blood glucose level. Managing the blood glucose level may support better eating habits and relationships with food. This must be assessed on a case-by-case basis through trial and error, as studies continue to show conflicting evidence concerning meal frequency and satiety.[103–106]

Now, probably the most overlooked factor, and one that supports us in the overall assessment of the client, is behavior. How does meal frequency affect behavior? And how does behavior affect meal frequency? We must consider the behavioral changes that come about through altered meal frequency.

Consider yourself for a moment. Think of a time when you were hungry, irritable, or your blood glucose was low. How did your perception of food change? Did you move toward less favorable foods or toward those that would solve the primary issue of blood glucose? Is this a conditioned response brought about by the repeated stimulus of timed eating patterns?[107] Is there an unconditioned response of salivation or an increase in stomach contractions around meal times that signify appetite? Consider your clients. If someone overconsumes calories regularly or makes poor choices by eating two meals a day, will consuming four meals change consumption and/or choices positively?

These are all questions we must consider when determining meal frequency. For many, an increase in meal frequency supports better emotional or behavioral responses surrounding food. It also means a level of conditioning that may move them away from old habitual patterns. Consider all aspects when deciding on meal frequency and remember that we can positively or negatively influence conditioning.

Summary

Decide on a meal frequency that is sustainable and syncs with the caloric intake an individual requires daily to achieve their goals. If their intake is high, consider increasing frequency to lower gastric stretch and to make meals more comfortable.

Note the individual's response to both higher and lower meal frequencies. Consider the behaviors affected. Having the client track behaviors and emotions in a food log may provide better answers.

Consider genetic factors and their phenotype, which may influence the individual's dietary habits and eating patterns associated with food choices. For example, if there are extended lengths of times between feedings, does this alter habits? We must differentiate between the need for food and the desire for food. For example, if a person skips breakfast and then walks past a bakery on the way to work, appetite (as opposed to hunger) results in the altered dietary patterns. If a person eats breakfast and then walks past a bakery, the sensory impact of the bakery is not as strong.

The need for food is an actual chemical alteration in the body brought about by a low level of glucose in the blood. This survival and protective response ensures adequate function of the body. As people manage and sustain glucose levels at different rates, we ask if it is indeed a physical need or simply a desire. We should also consider the rate and speed at which people eat. As different foods affect blood glucose differently and manage it at different levels, the latency between consumption and blood glucose signifying stability is adequate time for appetite to supersede hunger.

Appetite, unlike the physical reaction of hunger, is largely psychological. It can be a conditioned response (caused by the timings of meals, the environment, or feelings) or it can simply be impacted by senses. A good way to explain this is considering foods that do not look or smell great. Because of their appearance and aroma, the likelihood of overconsumption goes radically down. If you eat this unappealing food, you are satisfying appetite, not hunger. This is because that food did not influence the senses.

Therefore, if it smells great and looks great, it stimulates the involuntary physiological responses of salivation and stomach peristalsis (contractions) and makes you hungry. We will discuss this in more depth in chapter 13 when we look at the metabolic and satiety hormones.

CHAPTER 9: CALORIC DIFFERENTIALS

To understand the caloric model we are trying to build, we must understand the implications that occur when someone is put into a state of destructive (catabolic) or constructive (anabolic) metabolism. Remember, the goal in almost any compositional strategy is to maximize the result while minimizing the inevitable trade-offs.

The body is constantly striving for a level of homeostasis. Therefore, our intent is to push the body beyond its status quo. However we try to rework the conceptual patterns behind nutrition, it is irrefutable that the amount of total energy in and total energy out will remain the key determinants in total bodyweight.[108] This is irrespective of whether that total bodyweight presents itself as lean or fat mass.

In pursuit of lean muscular gain, and in hypercaloric states, we must therefore minimize lipogenesis and protein oxidation while looking to maximize protein synthesis. Anabolism means we are, in fact, stimulating net protein synthesis. In the pursuit of fat loss (lipolysis), and in a hypocaloric state, we must minimize the use of protein and amino acids as fuel (proteolysis).

Part of this equation is to minimize the acute and chronic adaptations brought about by both the hypo- and hypercaloric dieting environments. For example, someone at a clinically obese level wishing to lose body fat may work on a ratio of 3:1 of hypo- and hypercaloric levels. Someone looking to build lean tissue and maintain body fat may alternatively use a 1:3 ratio of hypo- and hypercaloric states. Remember that a hypocaloric state can also be brought about by an energetic output that is greater than intake. It is not solely a dietary model but one still in consideration of exercise and training.

Both environments, when approached chronically, will leave us with the inevitable residual trade-off. Managing how long we can spend in each state allows us to manage the physical state of the individual beyond the dated "bulk and cut" approach.

Through an in-depth understanding of the individual, their start point, and end goal, we can then determine the level of trade-offs necessary in this pursuit. When we discuss the trade-offs of extreme and rapid compositional changes later, this will be clearer.

The chronic or long-term implications of staying in either an energy surplus or deficit must be clear for us to understand not only the start point to an individual's strategy, but also how we relate this to the given time scale for change. The chronological dietary history can help us determine what metabolic changes, adaptations, or even dysfunctions may have occurred. The nutrients and foodstuffs that may have been dominating their dietary environment may be linked to poor behaviors surrounding those foods. This all must then be compiled and correlated to their current composition, end goals, and time scale.

This is a discussion point, not a generic point. There is no 12-week, 8-week, or similar plan that will get you from A to B. There is a plan that will move some toward a goal and others potentially past it. Your role as a coach is to look at all the factors, positive or negative, that play a part in the plan and from them, deduce the best course of action. For clients looking at extreme compositional changes, we must also verify the plan will be successful if we must pull someone back from a non-sustainable point and start them from a point that can successfully be sustained long term.

For example, I can take client A and client B from 15% body fat to 5% in two different time scales client A over 10 weeks and client B over 20 weeks. Assuming their start points are the same, the severity of what client A would need to do to get there lends no support to habitual changes. Everything they do is extreme: their caloric drop is steep. Their energy output is high fighting against a deficit for longer. They need to lose 1% body fat per week, whereas client B only needs to lose 0.5%.

Ask any client which they prefer. Ten weeks will win without a shadow of doubt. People want results tomorrow. This is where your skills as a coach, a businessperson, and an ethical human being come into play. At the point of client A's finish, there is a much higher level of metabolic deregulation than with client B. There is more extreme and uncomfortable food omittance within that time scale. The training regimen would be one that would be far less sustainable. The result following this state is, for many, catastrophic. Binge eating, loss of desire to train metabolically the body cannot handle the chronic intake that will now behaviorally occur. This is exactly what we are seeing a lot of in the modern era of extreme dieting. Impatience and extreme restrictions create irregular relationships with both food and exercise.

REVERSE PSYCHOLOGY

Three major principles surround reverse psychology that are worth noting: reactance, rebound, and curiosity.[109–111]

REACTANCE

When we are told we are forbidden something, we naturally feel threatened and that our freedom is being imposed upon. If I explicitly tell you that you are not permitted a particular food, psychology and studies tell us there is a higher likelihood you will seek it out.

REBOUND

"Try not to think about pizza." For those of you now salivating and feeling hungry, you are experiencing appetite, not hunger. Appetite is an involuntary physiological response and that phrase was enough to trigger it. Imagine muted responses from your satiety hormones and low blood glucose on top of that.

When we attempt to suppress a conscious thought, we productively think of things that in this case do not involve pizza. The responsive effect is that the thought becomes more insistent. Studies have revealed that suppression may be the starting point for obsession, rather than its initial intent. Many people we deal with divert a lack of control tangentially into a point of obsession. Others are already at that point and we may need to break down that obsession.

CURIOSITY

When there is a sign up saying, "Wet Paint," you inevitably want to touch it to see if the paint is wet. People become curious and intrigued when a restriction is imposed. Reactance and response are more relevant to the topic of nutrition, yet there may be times when people willingly alter nutritional strategies to try those that had positive results for a friend.

CALORIC INTAKE

To gain lean tissue, we must have a surplus of available "fuel" to do so. This must be heavily supported with a protein intake that is adequate for both cellular support and repair. To enable an increase in lean mass, we must first look to increase overall protein turnover to ensure protein synthesis nominally exceeds its breakdown. The more controlled breakdown we can achieve while still maintaining more synthesis, the faster we can ultimately acclimate to adaptive stimulus (training). For this to occur, we must be in an anabolic (regenerative) state and therefore hypercaloric state. We must also consider the aforementioned adaptive reserve and ensure the substrates that support it are also adequately supported.

To decrease body fat, lipolysis (the mobilization of fats for use as potential energy) must exceed lipogenesis (the storage of surplus energy substrates as subcutaneous fat). We must also be in a catabolic (degenerative) state. This can be enhanced somewhat by a lower level of plasma insulin and/or high catecholamines (stress hormones). This is achieved by lowering plasma glucose levels through a lower intake of carbohydrates around the training window or by an increased use of glycogen within training.

This culminates in an elevation of stress hormones, normally achieved by high-intensity training and/or the use of catecholamine-enhancing stimulants (such as caffeine) and allows fatty acids to be freed up to be potentially converted to energy. Preceding this with the sustained and elevated level of catecholamines and a lowered intensity of training allows these free and circulating fatty acids to be used as fuel. This is a discussion for my forthcoming training text, but from a nutritional standpoint, this is what we are largely striving for.

This is still overseen by the net amount of calories used against those taken in. You must still be hypocaloric to achieve a decreased body fat. This does become an issue when the metabolic hormones adjust to someone either taking in inadequate caloric intake for extended periods or simply expending too much energy.

It is a fine line between these two states: too long (and overly excessive) in one and you inherently gain fat, too long (and overly restrictive) in the other and you are likely to lose lean tissue. This is reflected by someone either exceeding or dropping below the hypothetical and ever-changing line of homeostasis.

Above the line in a hypercaloric state, the body has adaptive reserves; therefore, anabolism (regeneration) is possible without the catabolism (breakdown) of other stored metabolites. This is supported by the fact that, in a caloric surplus, the body also supports all relevant hormones that would increase this adaptive response to stimuli. Without sustaining this state, the breakdown and regeneration becomes much like spending more money than you earn. Everyday currency (energy substrates and hormones) must be supported beyond the spending that comes about through stress and stimulus (training and lifestyle).

Below the line in a hypocaloric state, the body is in a position in which it can use stored fuel as a resource. This could be from either stored or currently circulating levels of glycogen, amino acids, or fatty acids. Once depleted of muscle glycogen in a hypocaloric state, the body opts for its alternative: metabolites, protein, or fatty acids. The low blood glucose, coupled with high levels of stress hormones, bring about a survival response, which induces a breakdown of fatty acids that, once in circulation, can be used as fuel. Without this, amino acids or the body's own tissue will be sacrificed as fuel.

The goal in the pursuit of fat loss must be to do everything possible that is protective of lean tissue. This is one reason "show-level" dieting for natural unassisted athletes is generally longer than that of drug-assisted athletes. Assisted athletes preserve lean mass much better due to their enhanced level and their ongoing maintenance of a higher level of circulating hormones and increased adaptive reserve.

This is also why aggressive dietary restriction in non-assisted athletes has a far more profound impact on the circulating anabolic hormones in particular. Many of the rules we would apply to ectomorphic males, we can apply to female clients. Their circulating androgens are much lower; therefore, lean mass is compromised more.

Far too many people spend valuable time chasing the top line (mass gain or fat loss) instead of minimizing the inevitable cost. Composition is often a trade-off and we need to understand and consider that. Sometimes preventing fat gain and preventing muscle loss is a far easier strategy that aggressively trying to lower one or build the other.

DETERMINING INTAKE

The two most practiced methods to determine caloric intake are a standard basal metabolic rate (BMR) calculator and a food log. Readily available online, BMR calculators take your gender, height, weight, and activity level and provide a number based on this.

IMPERIAL BMR FORMULA

Women	BMR = 655 + (4.35 x weight in pounds) + (4.7 x height in inches) - (4.7 x age in years)
Men	BMR = 66 + (6.23 x weight in pounds) + (12.7 x height in inches) - (6.8 x age in years)

Women	BMR = 655 + (9.6 x weight in kilos) + (1.8 x height in cm) - (4.7 x age in years)
Men	BMR = 66 + (13.7 x weight in kilos + (5 x height in cm) - (6.8 x age in years)

HARRIS–BENEDICT FORMULA

Multiply your BMR by the appropriate activity factor to determine your total daily calorie needs:

If you are sedentary (little or no exercise)	BMR x 1.2
If you are lightly active (light exercise/sports 1–3 days/week)	BMR x 1.375
If you are moderately active (moderate exercise/sports 3–5 days/week)	BMR x 1.55
If you are very active (hard exercise/sports 6–7 days a week)	BMR x 1.725
If you are extra active (very hard exercise/sports & physical job or 2x training)	BMR x 1.9

The inherent flaw in this mathematical model is that it is based on very loose criteria, with no consideration for current or historical caloric intake.

For example, let's consider a serial female dieter. She is 80 kg (~176 lbs.), 170 cm (~5' 5"), and 30 years of age. Using a BMR calculator, her estimated intake should be 1588 k/cal daily. Because she is an avid gym member, this brings her estimated requirements up to 2739 k/cal.

Upon studying her comprehensive food log, it is apparent her average daily intake is around 1000 k/cal per day. This is not an uncommon discrepancy, but one in which the caloric deficit, in conjunction with the extent of exercise, would mean any weight loss would have resulted in not only a substantial amount of the desired fat loss, but a distinctly high ratio of loss from lean tissue and amino acid pools.

Our biggest issue alongside this is the number of adaptive metabolic changes that would have occurred to ensure survival: alteration in the HTPA axis, the autonomic nervous system, cytokines, and many other systems would have occurred. The result is a decrease in the anabolic, anorexigenic, and thermogenic hormones and an increase in the orixigenic and catabolic hormones. These serve to slow the rate of overall metabolic turnover, decreasing satiety hormones to signify hunger, and to up-regulate degeneration of tissue as fuel. What we would see is the perfect evolutionary response.

In a scenario such as this, the behavioral and psychological impact will be huge. Food and exercise will more than likely have obsessive tendencies and overly restrictive, and potentially binge-like, patterns.

The necessity to calculate calories is therefore redundant and gives little more than a loose starting point from which to determine a strategy. Some people, given no other direction, may make valuable use of such a mathematical tool as a starting point. This may not be optimal, but it is indeed a reference point.

The logic to simply log what you currently eat and then relate it to both bodyweight and/ or composition gives us a much clearer picture. Our largest issue to overcome is the noted underreporting of food intake in logs. Studies have shown levels of underreporting in both male and female populations.[108,112–115] As a coach, empathy and understanding surrounding current food choices is critical in the early stages of the client/coach relationship.

BMR also fails to acknowledge any type of metabolic dysfunction or chronic adaptation something we see a huge prevalence of in modern life that is a product of heredity, genetics, and the influential phenotype. Almost all issues revolve around abnormal levels of enzymes or hormones and, in some cases, the disorder of cells that absorb or function around the nutrients. There can also be potential build-ups of chemical mimickers that can disrupt the body's endocrine system. These can influence the number of hormone receptors in the body.

Change the amount of actual active hormones being produced. Block real hormones from accessing their receptors and influence the processing speed of these hormones. Despite these being "factors," the notion that these are major contributors to the health and obesity issues we are up against are speculative at best. Hormonal and metabolic adaptations are in constant flux: some we can manipulate through dietary means, but with others, the impact is minor.

Common metabolic dysfunctions we will see are hypo- and hyperthyroidism, which are indicative of an under- or overactive thyroid, respectively. The stages of beta-cell dysfunction are the progressive inability of the body to suitably secrete or manage insulin in response to a stimulus. If we reflect on the general societal approach to nutrition alongside the food industry's approach, it is no wonder these are common issues.

Chronic overexposure to the same foods over time, particularly those produced using non-traditional methods, can potentially culminate in an enzyme deficiency or simply a lack of basic supply over demand. This is common in Western society, where people have little variance in the types of food they eat.

Short-term abstinence from the "culprit" food and slow reintroduction in a controlled fashion is normally an adequate and effective solution. Secondary to this is when chemicals or medication damage the area where the enzyme is normally active, for example, in the small intestine. Observationally, I have found those with historical patterns of selective eating (being picky) tend to have more issues around the digestion and breakdown of food than others.

There is a belief in Western populations that gluten, wheat, and lactose appear to be the largest culprit foods and they have traditionally been chronically present within people's diets (think breakfast). There is much speculation behind the causes and issues, but there does appear to be solid rationalization in the quality of actual food and the ratio of gluten, enzymes, and bacteria within the food.

For example, fresh, traditionally made breads and pasta have much lower levels of gluten and higher levels of enzymes. Nations that use these foods as their staples seem to be much less exposed to issues with them. In comparison, processed versions of all of these foods have much higher ratios of gluten; therefore, over time, the exposure becomes much higher. Only in the case of those with celiac disease would complete omittance be required. In all other cases, short-term strategies can alleviate any symptoms. The sheer number of coaches omitting foods like these with no apparent reason is astounding and can cause the behavioral and habit issues previously mentioned.

One noted point is that when selective removal of foods or nutrients occurs, when that habit is broken, it is broken in abundance. Someone may "ban" themselves from refined sugars and put a time limit on it. When the target is reached or if the limit is broken it is highly likely that the nutrient or food is reintroduced at a binge level, not in mild or introductory amounts. This happens because of the negative response to the removal of the nutrient, not the nutrient itself. But sheer quantity reinforces the notion there is a reaction to that foodstuff.

Short-term omittance, in conjunction with inclusion of a good broad-spectrum plant enzyme and probiotic, may help with any of these intolerance symptoms. Dipeptidyl peptidase IV (DPP IV) appears to be promising with respect to gluten intolerance.

Both BMR and dietary log results are factors worth considering in the incremental or (as it is called for competitive physique athletes) "reverse" diet to establish the number of calories essential for function and to start again. Many serial dieters need to create stability in their patterns.

One thing you can guarantee is that anyone attempting to maintain a restrictive dieting pattern in both the nature and quantity of food will fail at some stage in the long term. Due to the aforementioned psychological reasons, this will generally be pretty momentous. Those with incredible amounts of psychological and physical fortitude may be the exceptions, or those with a relative short-term period of "dieting" as with physique athletes but they all once again remain on a tightrope between stable and inherently disordered eating patterns.

SUMMARY

There are many best practices a coach can implement to help clients manage caloric intake:

- Begin by establishing a level of empathy for current dietary habits and the forthcoming change that will be implemented from thorough and truthful reporting.
- Create a comprehensive dietary log of all food and drink.
- Monitor bodyweight at consistent times throughout the logging period (mornings are the most consistent).
- Review the average intake over the log period and determine if the TBM is increasing or decreasing given the caloric amount.
- Determine if current intake is reflective of the client's history.
- Review the client's goals and given timescales.
- Considering all this data, establish a baseline caloric intake and determine the level of flux you feel would move between an individual's hypo- and hypercaloric states in a safe manner.

Chapter 10: Metabolic Regulation and Metabolic Flux

Metabolic flux is the term used for the rate in which molecules and metabolites are turned over in a metabolic pathway. Metabolic regulation is the term used for the actions of food and transference into energy once ingested.

The three basic substrates we consume as energy are the macronutrients protein, carbohydrates, and fats. Through destructive metabolism brought about by the aforementioned hypocaloric state (a catabolic process), we can break these down into smaller molecules. This process can only be accomplished with the presence of the relevant enzymes; the term we use for this transference of energy is "metabolic regulation." This is the term used for the actions of food and its transference into usable energy once ingested.

Once broken down and digested, each substrate can be oxidized as fuel or stored as metabolic fuel (metabolites) for later use (based on demand) in the forms of either muscle glycogen (carbohydrate) or triacylglycerol (fat).

Both proteins and fats, metabolites obtained from dietary sources and the body's own stores, have capacity for secondary fuel usage. This is one of the many reasons that these will be statistically prioritized in any compositional diet. It is worth noting at this stage though that carbohydrates are protein-sparing, as they take responsibility for their primary role taking the burden off protein and fats. This offsets the necessity for the body to utilize other substrates as a secondary glucose provider. This is great if the preservation of lean mass or temporal elevation of certain metabolic hormones is a priority or a necessity. If fat loss is a priority this is counterproductive, so we run the risk then of lean tissue becoming compromised. Fluctuations between a glucose-fed state and one of depletion would be best served with most successful strategies.

This still always remains a calorie-driven model, but the fluctuations of protein and fats in a dietary strategy will be considerably less in most cases than that of carbohydrates, which we can use to manipulate energy systems easier.

During these processes, the energy released can be used or, as previously mentioned, stored as fuel by the muscle, fat, or liver cells. If the catabolic process of digestion is hindered, subsequently the availability of energy is also delayed. Anything that impairs digestion or absorption or indeed increases the endogenous loss will reduce the availability of immediate or sustained energy. Two people, therefore, on the same amount of macronutrients could be exposed to different amounts of usable energy available at different latency. The net amount though remains the same.

Because of the different thermodynamic properties of various macronutrients and the variance in efficiency, the notion that a calorie is a calorie means the laws of thermodynamics can be questioned.

Think of it like the bank putting a hold on your money. It is there, you just cannot spend it yet. It must be understood, however, that this does not detract from calories in versus calories out. It simply questions the timing of availability and an individual's efficiency in handling the substrate through its breakdown and absorption. It is often why you will observe different people responding at different stages to the same stimuli of nutrients.

NUTRIENT PARTITIONING

Throughout the entire process of metabolism, metabolic pathways dictate the body's requirements. In these different physiological states, nutrients and metabolic substrates are divided or partitioned between tissues and organs through the expression of enzymes and proteins specific to that particular tissue. An example is the one that provides the primary transport of glucose, GLUT-4.

GLUT-4 is found mainly in adipose tissue and striated muscle tissue (skeletal and cardiac). When insulin is present, it stimulates glucose uptake into these tissues by mobilizing GLUT-4 transporters from membranes within the cell to the membranes on the surface of the cell (plasma membrane).

This allows glucose from the bloodstream to bind to the GLUT-4 transporter and enter the cell. Declines in the insulin receptors that promote this uptake are hypothesized to be one of the major issues with insulin resistance. However, it is evident that in the presence of insulin resistance, the glucose and amino acids insulin may be carrying are unable to efficiently "upload" into the cell (like buffering on your computer). In the physique development world, this pathway needs to be efficient if we are to efficiently build lean tissue and positively alter body fat levels.

The body is like a mailroom, sending relevant substrates to relevant areas. To ensure the package arrives, it must have an efficient transporter. Upon arrival, the receptors must be welcoming or sensitive to the material. If not, the cells will be in a stage of resistance. In this case, the metabolic substrate will be forced to stay outside the cell, in the bloodstream, until such a stage that either it becomes welcoming or the substrate will be packed up as a stored metabolite.

This is also how insulin got its unnecessary bad reputation as a "storage hormone," as it does not just encourage the stimulation of GLUT-4 in muscle tissue but fat tissue also. A degree of insulin resistance means that the glucose that is unable to get into the cell has a high likelihood of being converted into fatty acids and becoming stored fuel. Insulin is not to blame, as it is simply doing its job.

Insulin resistance is brought about largely by poor and chronically poor dietary practices; therefore, this inefficient stage in partitioning must be brought up to speed by attempting to increase insulin sensitivity. The more efficient this becomes fundamentally, the easier it becomes to pack on muscle and keep body fat at bay. The leaner someone becomes, the more consistently efficient it also generally becomes.

Partitioning, much like the management and production of insulin, is very specific to the individual and is one of the fundamental reasons why diets can never be generic in nature. The subtle variations between human beings in both their genetic makeup and phenotype will influence the way in which substrates and calories are handled. If we consider the androgen levels of an individual alongside chronic catecholamine (stress) responses, each will respectively have an opposing effect yet be present at differing levels in an individual's phenotype and genotype.[96,116] We will discuss this in greater detail later, but two large factors are the presence of inflammatory markers.

Obesity, type 2 diabetes, and cardiovascular disease appear to share the same metabolic environment as insulin resistance and this chronic subacute inflammation.[117]

At this stage, we could get engrossed in the scientific intricacies of these interactions. What we fundamentally aim to accomplish, aesthetically, with the majority of our clientele will give us the welcome by-product of decreased inflammation we desire.

"Many dietary practitioners act like school kids playing sports. They run around aimlessly chasing the ball, when often the ball will come to them if they just think intelligently about their strategy and implement it accordingly."

~Phil Learney

Through the lowering of both subcutaneous and visceral compartments of fat, increasing overall activity levels, and the improvement of dietary practices, the sequela shows improved insulin sensitivity, reduced inflammatory markers, and a lowered risk of cardiovascular disease. Beyond these welcome by-products, we are undoubtedly looking at medical intervention that is beyond our scope of practice.

In nutrient partitioning, we must also consider the physiological parameter that dictates the compartmentalization of fluid and its individual variability. Fluid can be broadly subdivided into two types: intracellular fluid (ICF) and extracellular fluid (ECF). These amass 60–65% and 35–40% of the body's water respectively.

Electrolyte concentration, blood circulation, and metabolism of tissue will all be factors in these levels. When considering electrolytes, sodium and potassium in particular will play active roles in these ratios, as they are partly responsible for transporting fluid into cells (think osmosis). The areas of concern here will be the level of sodium in processed foods and perhaps a lack of good quality sodium within the regular diet.

Again, in reference to salt, we are once again up against a generic demonizing of a critical component of an individual's diet. The use of high-quality non-refined salts within a non-processed diet is generally a good practice.[118] The physical appearance of an individual may well be influenced by this and when considering more complex nutritional strategies these should be considered; however, they are beyond the realm of this particular text.

A key element missing from even the most basic of nutritional strategies, particularly when considering training, is the inclusion of electrolytes and hydration. In and around the workout window, consuming fluid and electrolytes can serve to assist neural communication between cells and overall cellular recovery. The distribution of sodium (Na+) and potassium (K+) across these different compartments plays a role in polarization and the membrane potential of cells.

CALORIC RESTRICTION (HYPOCALORIC)

Any caloric restriction will result in weight loss if energy intake is lower than expenditure it is that simple. Caloric restriction means that, inevitably, we will be in a state of catabolism or destructive metabolism. This is the basic state required o attain fat loss, but it is detrimental to lean muscle mass if we chronically remain in this state. The body goes through a series of necessary metabolic adaptations to ensure overall survival in such a state. If we did not have this compensatory mechanism, it would inevitably result in malnourishment and then death. Energy and fat stores are protected by a series of bioenergetic and neurobiological physiologies what we call adaptive thermogenesis.[119]

During this process, the body goes through a series of baseline homeostatic adaptations to preserve energy. The human body is constantly striving for homeostasis. In any dietary approach, when the body has a surplus of energy, we are in what is classed "constructive metabolism" (anabolism). Basically, this means there is adequate fuel to repair and fuel the body beyond its normal requirements.

Alongside this, we see a supporting rise in both the anabolic and metabolic hormones. In direct contrast, in a caloric deficit, we see a rise in catabolic hormones, initiating the process of destructive metabolism brought about by a hypocaloric state. In this case, we are the position where the body will break down its own stores of metabolites as fuel those it deems both efficient in breakdown and surplus to fundamental requirements. All fairly simple, right? Just basic physiological survival.

In both states, we have relative trade-offs. In any hypercaloric state, we run the risk of fat gain; in a hypocaloric state, there is the risk of lean tissue loss. Therefore, we must grasp that any chronic or long-term period in either state becomes detrimental to almost all physique- or performance-oriented goals. The exception perhaps being when body mass is negative to requirements and it is just simply better to be at a lower bodyweight, even at the detriment of muscle tissue.

Putting together a strategy for fat loss or muscle gain is often down to selecting the quantifiable periods of time someone would be required to spend above or below the hypothetical line of homeostasis. Consistency is key, but if a nominal amount of calories keeps you in a state of restriction, the cost long term of a degree of lean tissue loss must be accounted for. Offsetting this is the key and will be determined by the degree of trade-off for an individual's personal goals or physique.

As a coach, one of the decisions we are left with is the time scale in which someone has to achieve their desired goals. The industry and fitness media has positioned us with very generic timescales when it comes to physique transformations. The 12-week transformation seems all too common and shorter versions appear out of the necessity and their inherent sales value of being shorter in time. Everyone wants results yesterday.

Note what it takes for someone to diet and make a series of uncomfortable changes to their lives in a period as short as eight weeks. And not only that, but also achieve results. Both their training and diet will undoubtedly run them into the ground and the inevitable cost to metabolism will only be to their detriment over the long term. In later chapters, we will discuss the homeostatic changes that occur when these non-sustainable and aggressive approaches are taken.

After their eight-week program, what is the last thing they want to do? Continue? What about all the foods they undoubtedly took pleasure from that you banned them from consuming? They are tired and worn out, their libido is shot, they look a little leaner, and they have removed themselves from social circles all of which are things they took pleasure from. Behaviors are ingrained and the psychological understanding of why changes were made has had insufficient time to be fully understood and validated.

The trade-off is some nice pictures of them with abs, a dysfunctional metabolism, a dysfunctional relationship with food, and a social circle that perhaps needs a little TLC. In response, as you have taken away their freedom of choice, they now progress to consuming everything they have missed or felt deprived of. They now have a hatred of working out and want to socialize heavily to reignite friendships. It runs deeper than this, as mentioned earlier in the text, but hopefully, you are starting to understand the trade-offs better. The leaner someone wishes to become, the more behaviors and habits need to change.

You, as an individual or company, have just lost that person as a client under the hope that the uncomfortable experience you just put them through will draw them back again. There is a chance that once they gain back all the weight and want to do it again, they will. Ethical, right? You can answer that.

> *"Don't give people fish . . . teach them to fish."*
> *~Old Adage*

We are responsible for not only people looking good for a moment, but for helping be able to sustain a healthy and happy body image long term: to make training enjoyable, to ensure that food is seen not only as fuel, but also as something that can be enjoyed. The ability of a coach to honestly assess how long it will take someone to get from A-B and then be able to sustain it is a skill that likely cannot be taught.

The understanding of cost and extreme physique changes relies on distinct differentials between those that use hormonal assistance versus those that do not. Those that may have more genetically suited physiques yield better to fat loss and lean tissue maintenance or gain. Those using hormonal assistance or with better genes would have a shorter time scale to achieve what someone slightly less genetically superior can achieve.

When someone says, "Can I do that?" the answer would be a series of "depends" and "buts," based on not only what the individual is prepared to give but what their body is capable of giving.

When put into a hypocaloric state, the body adjusts the HTPA axis, autonomic nervous system, cytokines, and other systems. Long-term caloric restriction does not just simply act like a "fuel in, fuel out" scenario: it alters the way in which fuel is inherently managed. Different people will have altering efficiency in these management options depending upon a great deal of dietary history.

Through the reduction of calories, we create a void in requirements, thus the body will use whichever metabolite is most available as a way in which to fuel itself. This is basic economy and can be seen much like in biomechanics. When moving a weight from A to B, the body will take the most efficient pathway when underload. Our understanding of metabolic function will allow us to manipulate the scenarios that occur through altering nutritional and potentially training variables.

At this stage, we must be aware of the aforementioned genetic factors.[120] It has been hypothesized that bodyweight and composition of an individual is dependent upon four factors: food intake, nutrient turnover, thermogenesis, and level of adiposity.[121]

This brings about the notion of the set point and the fact that the genetic physiology of an individual (regardless of current composition) will play a role in their management, partitioning, and regulation of nutrients. Knowing the history of a client can give us great clues with respect to their predispositions.

In a calorie-restricted (CR) diet, individuals display variance in the way both protein and fat is mobilized for use and non-exercise activity thermogenesis (NEAT). The body always has reserves of body fat and protein for use as energy. In any kind of energy restriction, the body, based on numerous physiological factors, will determine this ratio of usage and the type of metabolic adaptation.

We are always erring on the side of muscular preservation, as when an individual loses body fat, lean muscle mass typically decreases concomitantly over time at slowing rates.

Eston[122] found that in six weeks of a very-low-calorie diet (VLCD), 63% of weight loss was from fat and the remaining 37% was from FFM. Other studies have shown similar statistics. There is clear evidence that the degree of caloric restriction and rate of weight loss affect the percentage loss of FFM in hypocaloric diets.[123–126]

Resistance training has been shown to help preserve lean mass during hypocaloric dieting.[127–129] Several metabolic adaptations also occur to preserve muscle mass. In periods of starvation or caloric restriction, secretion of thyroid hormones decreases. This is thought to be caused by the decrease in leptin and its concurrent impact on the hypothalamic release of TSH.

Put simply, the more fat someone has when starting a diet, the higher ratio of fat will be used as fuel in the onset. The less fat someone has, the more the body will favor a higher ratio of protein. Conversely, the higher the level of adiposity when put into an overfed state, the more fat will be stored and less lean mass gained. The leaner the individual, the more protein will be stored (LBM gain) and less fat stored.

Someone who is naturally lean will typically have a high NEAT, a better ratio of fat mobilization and usage in a hypocaloric state (due to genetic factors), and better protein storage capacity in a fed state (think testosterone and its protective abilities). Someone who has "dieted" to get lean still has the same base genetic profile. Their body is still primed like someone with naturally high body fat. The moment they move from dieting to an overfed state, the body will store more in fat compartments. In contrast, naturally lean individuals will gain more lean mass and store less fat.

This reiterates the importance of knowing the dietary and physiological history of someone in order to put together not only an initial strategy but also a long-term maintenance strategy. When we discuss reverse dieting later in this chapter, this will also come into play. We will discuss the inherent flaws in different strategies and the chronic misuse of even the most effective strategies, but for now, the focus will primarily be on CR and the manipulation of carbohydrates.

It is clear that any form of caloric restriction for prolonged periods creates numerous homeostatic adaptations. Adaptive thermogenesis will result in a decrease of total daily energy expenditure (TDEE), reduction in exercise activity thermogenesis (EAT), and reduction in NEAT. Alongside this, there will also be an increase in mitochondrial efficiency.[109,130–146]

In some people, over several weeks of caloric restriction, there is also an increase in the lipoprotein lipase (LPL) enzyme. This is responsible for removal of lipids from the blood and into storage. Fat storage therefore becomes enhanced when normal eating is resumed. We discuss the adjustments of NEAT, TDEE, and the thyroid further in chapter 13.

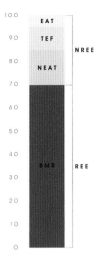

Figure 7 Components of daily energy expenditure.

CALORIC SURPLUS (HYPERCALORIC)

In the pursuit of a dynamic and goal-specific balance between a state of tissue regeneration or degeneration, we must not only grasp the ratio of time spent in each metabolic state, but also the frequency required to elicit the planned goal and the required rate of weight loss or gain. This must carefully consider the trade-off offs that would inevitably be encountered and the altered relationship with food that will undoubtedly occur.

In the case of hypercaloric diets, much like hypocaloric diets, the degree of caloric increase or restriction will affect the percentage of fat mass gained in surplus or the amount of FFM lost in deficit. The steeper the increment, the higher the percentage; therefore, long-term sustainability will be questioned. Patience in compositional change becomes something that will support and stabilize the longevity of change. However, this will probably never detract from the client's demand for results now.

In any hypercaloric diet, increases in muscle mass and fat mass can, and in most cases do, occur. The somewhat dated concept of the "bulk" phase revolves around the acceptance of this inevitable increase in fat mass. The rationale is that when someone would move from this excessive hypercaloric state, the gained muscle will be kept but the fat associated with a "cut" or proceeding hypocaloric state will be lost. This approach was largely popularized by assisted bodybuilders who offset the drop in anabolic and metabolic hormones through their exogenous administration while chronically staying in a hypocaloric state in the cutting phase.

For unassisted bodybuilders or those pursuing positive compositional changes, the bulk/cut approach as a block-periodized method is effective yet riddled with poor trades in metabolic function. A planned undulating approach based on initial composition will show far greater and more sustainable results in the case of both assisted and non-assisted physique athletes. This will be discussed in detail later.

Forbes[117] theorized a framework trying to predict the level and ratio of compositional change in relation to FFM and FM. It was first seen that leaner individuals saw a greater increase in lean tissue than that of obese people by up to 30% over a 3-week hyperenergetic diet. There are huge questions regarding this model and others have conversely assumed a constant state of weight loss or gain.[147–151]

There are far too many variables both from a hormonal and nutritional standpoint to generally theorize a model for an accurate predictive weight loss. The homeostatic adaptations that occur in both hyper- and hypoenergetic diets must therefore be considered and accounted for alongside the physiological status of the individual before embarking on any plan. By understanding the homeostatic adaptations that occur both chronically and acutely, we can minimize negative trade-offs and plan effective strategies alongside a theorized and individualized prediction of weight loss.

Much like in caloric restriction, many homeostatic adaptations occur in a caloric surplus:[117,142,152–158]

- Increase in insulin levels and insulin sensitivity (decrease in blood fatty acid concentrations)
- Increase in GH, IGF-1, and free and total testosterone [unbinds from sex hormone binding globulin (SHBG)]
- Increase in thyroid uptake and conversion
- Decrease in catecholamine response, adrenaline, noradrenaline, ACTH, cortisol, and glucagon, which causes a reduction in catecholamine-induced lipolysis and a reduction in the amount of glucose produced by the liver
- Decrease in ghrelin levels
- Increase in leptin levels
- Increase in muscle and fat mass
- Increase in protein synthesis

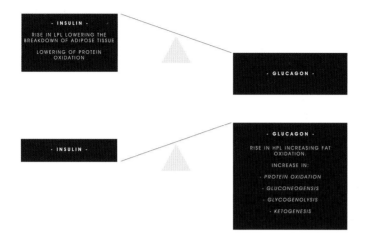

Figure 8 The balance between levels of insulin and glucagon.

Through the decrease of carbohydrates, we influence the levels of insulin and blood glucose. This decrease is essential if we are to look at fat loss as opposed to simply weight loss. A lowered level of insulin alongside a lowered concentration of glucose in the blood means we have an increased rate of both proteolysis (the breakdown of protein) and lipolysis (breakdown of fat) largely due to glucagon concomitantly rising.

Glucagon acts on the liver, allowing stored glycogen and amino acids to be converted into glucose (glycogenolysis and gluconeogenesis, respectively). It also stimulates, in the right scenario, the breakdown of fatty acids into ketone bodies (ketogenesis). Probably the biggest factor given the topic is its action upon adipose cells. It stimulates lipolysis, the breakdown of fatty acids into usable fuel, which is critical if fat loss is the goal.

In contrast, a rise in levels of insulin brings about the reduction and inhibition of glucagon. It stimulates uptake of glucose into cells (thus lowering blood glucose), increasing positively both metabolism and anabolism.

Insulin and glucagon work in unison to keep circulating blood glucose at adequate levels. Many people, despite these regulatory systems being in place, struggle to adapt to the change in metabolic pathways. Most Westerners are carbohydrate-adapted; therefore, they function far more efficiently when insulin acts as the main regulator of fuel. For many, this will be an accessible and easily used fuel source. Glucagon, in most cases, is far more inefficient. In all cases, adaptation takes time and sometimes includes a respective trade-off.

When we consider the demographics, it must be understood that these fundamental processes are often compromised through various mechanisms. This leads to a degree of what is commonly known as metabolic inflexibility.

METABOLIC FLEXIBILITY

Metabolic flexibility is the term used to indicate an individual's ability to switch fuel sources seamlessly and efficiently under varying nutritional conditions: the ability largely to move between the use of amino acids or lipids as fuel in the absence of adequate glucose. It is commonly referred to as people being "fat-adapted" or "carb-adapted."

This is the exact scenario most individuals want to be in. The flexibility in their diet is reflective of the flexibility surrounding metabolic pathways. This is why the notion that flexible dieting or fitting your macros simply will not work effectively for most of the general populous. Those that popularize these methods disregard, or are inattentive to, the present metabolic condition of the individual.

Individuals displaying a good physiological condition can and will have success with flexible approaches to dieting. Some coaches transfer what they have had personal success with directly to their metabolically compromised clientele with a distinct disregard for the reinforcement of better behaviors. A simple "can" or "can't" regarding food seems to be a perpetuated topic instead of the outcome of different dietary choices in conjunction with its impact on physiology, behavior, and preexisting habits.

There is a significant relationship between obesity, insulin resistance, and metabolic inflexibility. Metabolic flexibility is impaired in type 2 diabetic subjects; therefore, the linear degradation in glucose management coincides with this adjustment.[159]

Lean and cardiovascular individuals in a fasted state have a high reliance on fat oxidation. In a fed, insulin-stimulated state, the lean individual suppresses fat oxidation flawlessly and moves to a high rate of glucose usage. However, in the obese population, fat oxidation is poorly suppressed and there is significantly less stimulation of glucose oxidation.

This fundamentally means that any degree of obesity incrementally slows the switch between fat to glucose oxidation (metabolic inflexibility). In lean individuals, this ability is highly efficient (metabolically flexible).[160–164]

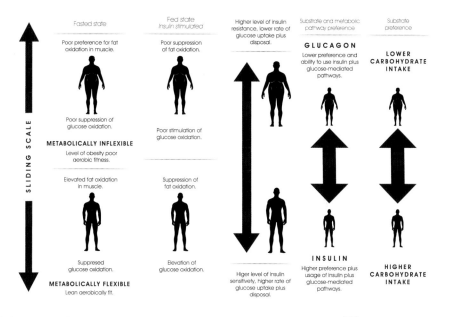

Figure 9 Substrate and metabolic pathway preference: adapted from Kelley.[171]

Conversely, lean individuals show a greater propensity toward using carbohydrates as fuel (glycolysis) in insulin-stimulated or "fed" conditions and thus suppress lipid oxidation. Therefore, due to numerous factors, the leaner someone is, the less important fuel quality is. Thus, the inclusion of "dirty foods" can be more frequently consumed with minimal or no consequence. Make note that alongside the digestion, absorption, and assimilation of carbohydrates improving, their ability to switch between substrate use is heightened and undoubtedly one of the by-products is a more efficient and healthier digestive system.

Metabolic flexibility is, in essence, the body's ability to switch between the insulin- and glucagon-mediated pathways and the surrounding elements of nutrient assimilation supporting this. Kelley and Mandarino defined metabolic flexibility as "the capacity to switch from predominantly lipid oxidation and high rates of fatty acid uptake during fasting conditions to the suppression of lipid oxidation and increased glucose uptake, oxidation, and storage under insulin-stimulated conditions."[172]

Establishing the flexibility of the body to move into the "starved" conditions of gluconeogenesis as opposed to the "fed" conditions of glycolysis is critical for many in long-term dietary success. As mentioned, many people are simply inefficient at this switch from glycolysis (stimulated by insulin) to gluconeogenesis (stimulated by glucagon). This is why people find switching from heavy .

carbohydrate diets to largely protein and fats difficult. This is largely due to the resultant hypoglycemia that will occur prior to adaptation and the often-aggressive approach toward the often unnecessarily aggressive lowering and prolonged approach to carbohydrates.

Almost all foods we consume are insulinogenic, meaning that, in response to ingestion, there is a rise in the production of insulin by the beta cells in the pancreas. Under fasting conditions, or in the absence of insulin, the body will switch from glycolysis to gluconeogenesis through the release of glucagon by the pancreatic alpha cells. This release initiates the catabolic action of gluconeogenesis and the concurrent generation of glucose from non-carbohydrate sources including pyruvate, lactate, glycerol, and amino and fatty acids.

Remember that catabolism is an essential function and something people spend too long dwelling on as a problem (they also do this in the case of cortisol, which is ironically the initiator of gluconeogenesis). It will also elicit the catecholamine-induced lipolysis and force the liver to produce more glycogen.[165]

Gluconeogenesis permits us to transport amino acids, either from a surplus dietary pool or from our body's own tissue (storage) to be converted to glucose. This is a rudimentary survival response and the reason we should reduce caloric numbers and the pool of carbohydrates responsible for glycolysis. We must increase the pool of available amino acids if muscle preservation is a goal.

Insulin is a pancreatic peptide hormone central in metabolic regulation. It acts in many ways: regulating blood sugar, elevating protein synthesis (proteogenesis), inhibiting the breakdown of fats (lipolysis), and stimulating the uptake of glucose into both lean and fatty tissue.

REVERSE DIETING

Now here comes the hard sell. The period after restrictive dieting is when your body is most primed to quickly grow lean tissue and keep fat loss to a minimum. You have made the things that dropped in response to caloric restriction hypersensitive to its elevation (think refeeding, but with a long-term impact). As previously mentioned, studies have shown that a large amount of metabolic hormones, particularly the thyroid hormones, can be elevated through hypercaloric dieting and increased carbohydrate intake.[166]

This concept is not just one we can apply to contest dieting or those pursuing extreme fat loss. This is also relevant to the clientele many of us will, or have been, dealing with. Chronic or yo-yo dieting, in whatever form, leaves a footprint. That historical footprint gives us a lot of the information required to alter any negative metabolic effects that may have occurred. A lot of nutrition is logical in hat when substrates need to be manipulated, the negative manifestations that have occurred through either excess or omittance of them is often counteracted when reintroduced at the opposing, yet regulated, level. What was once low and had negative impact when elevated can help reverse this.

After a period of linear or non-linear caloric or substrate restriction, there will be the aforementioned and discussed alterations to metabolic physiology. Again, the steeper this restriction path, the more negative implications will occur physiologically and behaviorally. Now, understanding the concept of both refeeding and what chronic or short-term changes would have occurred, we can develop a better understanding of how to successfully reset the body to a point when there are not negative health implications or fat gain.

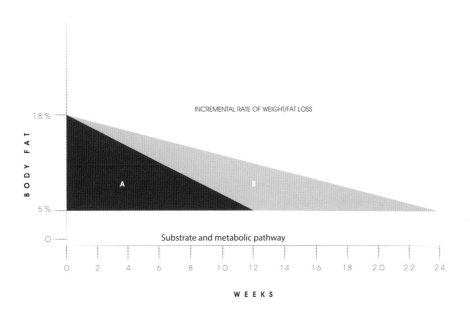

Figure 10 Diagram of steep increments.

Figure 10 shows the incremental rate of fat loss. The steeper the increment and more severe the rate of loss, the lower the likelihood of sustainable management is. The severity of changes that accompany these accelerated processes are often physically, mentally, and behaviorally unsustainable. The competing behaviors will also come into alignment with former physiological states. Someone who has been compositionally sound needs to make very few and minimal alterations to currents habits, behaviors, lifestyle, and diet. For obese populations, the severity of change will be dramatic

At a given state in reverse dieting (if we wish to use that term), you must determine if a series of systems are either up- or down-regulated. Let's take the basic case of a bodybuilder. Understandably, there can be several approaches, but, in general, there will have been a reduction in overall calories throughout the process. There will have also have been a reduction in carbohydrates. Fats and protein will have more than likely been elevated to alleviate potential lean tissue loss.[167–172]

The reversal process is no more complicated than the increase in both carbohydrates and calories over a period of time when attempting to establish a maintainable level of calories, carbohydrates, proteins, and fats all of which attempt to maintain a sustainable compositional level that is conducive with health and lifestyle.

We know very little at present beyond largely hypothesized incremental rates of elevation. Again, we are possibly seeking a mathematical model or set number instead of perhaps an individual and sensible approach relative to feedback.

I hope that from what we have learned thus far, we can grasp that the steeper, more aggressive, and restrictive the change in energetic intake, output, and food choices, the higher the likelihood that the proceeding behaviors become both dysfunctional and non-sustainable. Also, the notion of simply "sucking it up" and temporally dealing with the behavioral, social, and habitual fallout leads to negative results. Following a period of dieting, there is a high chance of not only a degree of metabolic dysfunction, but also a negative and detrimental change in the way food, its relationship to function, and body image are viewed.

We must remember we are influencing psychology, behaviors, and habits. Good coaches will be able to grasp the respective trade-offs, discuss them with the client, and thoroughly consider the long game as opposed to just simply the short-term effects.

CHAPTER 11: SET-POINT THEORY

The set-point theory suggests that through a series of homeostatic and biological controls, the body is regulated between a narrow set of self-regulated parameters. Bodyweight and body fat, in this case, are regulated by a series of biological feedback loops and mechanisms that control caloric intake and storage compartments.[173,174]

There are only a select few variables, but the set point supports a narrow range in which the body will self-regulate bodyweight, adipose tissue, compartments of fluid, and much more. The genetic effect of DNA, epigenetics, or heritability combined with environmental effects and phenotype result in the product of bodyweight. This supports the hypothesis that we are genetically predisposed yet, over time, through phenotype, slowly adjusting or influencing this set point (also called "settling point").

For many who have repeated effective dietary protocols over numerous years or phases, they will note a similar phenomenon that slowly allows the body to adopt a better set-point composition.[175] In contrast, it appears that those who have been subject to poor dietary practices see a resulting negative influence on satiety signaling and the disruption in communication between these biological control systems.

"Obesity seems to be perpetuated by a series of vicious cycles which, in combination with increasingly obesogenic environments, accelerate weight gain and represent a major challenge for weight management."
~Swinburn and Egger[84]

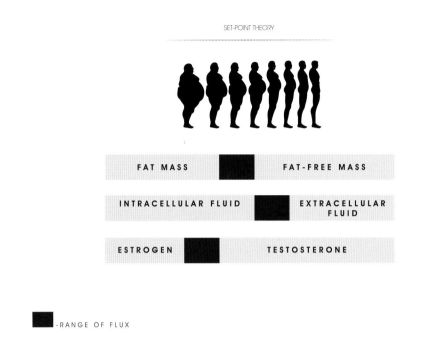

Figure 11 The set-point theory would support a narrow flux in which physiological levels of various components range. The level of extracellular and intracellular compartmentalization of fluid will make one physique look dramatically different from the next.

Worldwide, on a genetic level, the human being is going through incredibly slow evolutionary adaptations. If we then consider the set point and the influence environment and dietary choices have had in the past in even the past century this influence is observationally apparent.

We no longer eat for survival, but for satisfaction, pleasure, and other social and habitual reasons. Compounded with the array of foods now designed and presented to not only satiate hunger but to aggressively stimulate appetite, we can see why this set point is generally moving negatively across the population.

If all has been successful with the initial dietary approach, the body is at the stage in which it will be using fatty acids for energy incredibly efficiently and will have adapted within the proportionate caloric deficit. If suitable amino acid levels have been maintained to support androgens, peptides, and the positive synthesis of protein, muscle loss will be at a minimum. At this point, the body will be in a heightened state of metabolic elevation and flexibility.

The goal must be to elevate calories steadily out of a deficit while capitalizing on the elevated metabolic rate. This means we can add calories into the diet up to the maintenance level until body fat levels begin to rise. It is a fine line and one that cannot be determined by a static mathematic equation. The proportional rate and increment of calories are also tricky to determine and, given what we know, are merely hypotheses right now.

Personally, I attempt, in most cases, to bring up calories to maintenance as quickly and as comfortably as possible. At this stage, the gastric system may be a little less tolerant of food quantity so conferring with the client and making decisions based on feedback is a much better approach.

It would be expected in the CR phase that androgens and thyroid hormones would have declined. In addition to this, plasma insulin would have decreased, but cellular sensitivity would have positively increased, as would the level of glucagon being released by the alpha cells. Cortisol is also more than likely to be raised with other catecholamines (particularly if stimulants have been used at later stages of dieting).

Thyroid stimulus will be somewhat self-managed, as the incremental increase in calories should create an adequate steady stimulus to up-regulate them back to basal levels. Elevation of dietary fats is in support of androgen production. Studies have shown that diets containing ~20% fat, compared with a diet containing ~40% fat, show significant reductions in testosterone. The replacement of dietary carbohydrates with proteins has also been shown to decrease testosterone concentrations.[176–181]

Reintroducing carbohydrates and fats incrementally while moving the elevated protein levels down to maintenance level would be supportive of all the down-regulated systems while capitalizing on the extra sensitivity brought about through the dieting phase.

THE PARADIGM OF CLEAN EATING

We have mentioned several times how we need to understand the implications of dietary methods and modalities and how they affect different people for different reasons.

Flexible dieting, macro counting, or "if it fits your macros" (IIFYM) are currently popular. Now, if we were looking for a system that regulates caloric intake while ensuring adequate macronutrients are available for repair, we have it therein. Provided the programming is adequate, this is ideal and ultimately very sustainable in many respects. However, it still has potential to become a compulsion or disorder for many. Feeling the necessity to allocate everything that passes their lips in a log or digital app can lead us to better self-regulation, which is what many need.

However, this can develop into an equally unhealthy compulsion such as eating chicken and broccoli six times a day. Creating a self-regulatory environment with occasional returns to controlled patterns to simply ensure things are kept orderly is a better psychological and behavioral approach. In today's world of food, and the clever way in which food is marketed, I feel these frequent revisits to assess intake are inevitable necessities for most people.

Now, if we are to understand this better, we must walk a moment in someone else's shoes. The discussion, or perhaps argument, in the industry continues to reign between clean and flexible eating. In many respects, people are arguing about the wrong thing, as usual. There appears to be a necessity to belong to a camp or method and this is where perspective comes in handy.

We spoke earlier about the difference between hunger and appetite. We will also cover satiety and metabolic hormones later in the text, But for now, let's simply look at food and the behaviors that surround it.

Earlier, we discussed the need to be aware of "trigger" foods foods people struggle to regulate intake of or resonate toward for a multitude of reasons. Someone who is lean and somewhat content physically has, by default, a regulated and functional signaling mechanism for blood glucose and satiety coming from their specific regulators (insulin, glucagon, ghrelin, and leptin primarily). This is where we must consider false hunger and again must understand the difference between hunger and appetite.

Hunger, as noted, is a physical reaction in response to low blood glucose, thus signaling a chemical response. This initiates hunger signals to ensure the body gets the nutrients it requires to function.

If someone with any type of metabolic dysfunction (again, generally the higher level of obesity, the more prevalent this typically becomes with the exception of metabolic benign obesity), the management of blood glucose is poor. Therefore, "false hunger" occurs. The body signals hunger and the notion it is in need of energy when, in fact, the signaling is just poor.

The leaner someone is, the better this signal classically becomes. When you also consider the psychology, the reduction in social pressure, and potential change in mood this brings about, it is clear this is a much more manageable situation.

"Just Eat Less"

Appetite is a sensory or psychological reaction to food that stimulates salivation and stomach contractions, both of which are involuntary. This is what we experience when we smell something good or see something appetizing.

Now let's consider the flexible and potentially self-regulated approach we are striving for with someone who is both at a level of metabolic dysfunction and psychologically unhappy with the way they look. To compound this, we can almost be sure the behaviors and habits surrounding food are much stronger and more frequent than those who sustain a much leaner physique and are happier with their appearance.

For example, place a pizza in front of this person. (Pizza typically comes in multiple serving sizes, not just one. Almost all foods generically serve two or more; very few are single portion.) Tell this person they are only allowed two slices to hit their macronutrient or caloric requirement. Will they be compliant? This depends.

Pizza is calorie-dense, so two slices are ingested fast. The blood glucose has not had adequate time to rise. However, even with dysfunctional management, the signal perhaps has not had adequate time to register that blood glucose is moving toward a stable level. Therefore, they still have a hunger signal. The pizza looks good and smells great. Appetite now kicks in so they have a myriad of strong signals urging them to eat another slice.

They are psychologically and physically not in a good place right now and they often do not care one bit if it blurs their nonexistent muscular definition, as the temporal satisfaction it will provide is an immediate reward. They have behaviors and past habits that also influence this decision. Perhaps they have never eaten only one slice before. Or they may even perceive financial loss from not eating it all.

Now I ask again, "Will they be compliant?" Would clean food less appetizing, with a less tantalizing aroma or fewer behaviors attached to it have made them more compliant? Would exchanging the pizza slice for something without an excess of calories have been successful? Could I have given them a burger or something pleasurable in exchange?

Something that comes as a single portion is generally preferable. By the time they received a second portion, hunger would be satiated and they would not want it. This is where the analogy about waiting before ordering dessert comes from. You satiate hunger and the dessert is not in front of you, so you end up perhaps not ordering it. But what if you order it straight away? Blood glucose has had less time to stabilize and when dessert arrives, it creates the involuntary salivating and stomach contractions. You end up eating it based on appetite, not hunger.

"WE MUST DEFINE THE DIFFERENCE BETWEEN NEEDS AND WANTS"

We must think not only about the types of food but we must also understand that person's physiological position. To broadly prescribe any dietary system while ignoring someone's physiological and psychological stage is unwise.

If you give a metabolically and behaviorally dysfunctional person a pack of biscuits and tell them to eat only two, you have imposed a restriction (look back to reverse psychology). You are also dealing with someone that cannot just eat two biscuits. The food creates pleasure and makes them happy, but it will not influence hunger signals, so these signals remain and the sensory response means appetite is thriving. If we could buy biscuits individually, perhaps we could avoid this. But then again, perhaps but we couldn't.

Chapter 12: Nutrient Cycling, Shifting, and Loading

The human body is a mix of altering variables: the digestive, circulatory, immune, endocrine, nervous, lymphatic, and muscular systems all coexisting, communicating, and adapting to one another. These adaptations are brought about by our altered environment, external stimulus, stressors, and a major factor the nutrients we ingest.

The strategic and non-strategic fluctuations of macronutrients and/or calories are expected in any regular diet. However, we can take advantage of controlling the inherent variability within a diet and placing some form of advantageous structure around it. Most of these systematic approaches serve to take advantage of the metabolic changes that occur in a shorter acute term.

Carb cycling, carb back-loading, fasting in all of its guises, cheats, refeeds, and caloric shifting are all terms we are familiar with. But what purpose do they all serve?

There is the somewhat hypothetical notion that "keeping the body guessing" is the best way to ensure any type of physical progression. But this, in many respects, goes against the basis of adaptation. There is very little that is adapted to by the body in such an acute way that after a meal or a workout, the body will "switch" to immediately accommodate for it in some way.

CALORIES

Probably the first thing we can consider is calories. We must consider what we have already learned about hyper-, hypo-, and isocaloric dieting and the difference and variability between constructive and destructive metabolism.

Inevitably, if we spend too long in a destructive state, over time, we will lose a ratio of lean muscle mass alongside body fat. The more extreme the diet, the more unfavorable this ratio is likely to become. Too long in a constructive state and we will invariably, alongside the development of tissue, accumulate surplus body fat as part of the process of storing fuel. Again, the degree of extremity largely mediates this and guides us back to the notion and practice of bulking phases.

The obvious initial point when determining any level of intake is to decide which goal is the priority: to build lean mass, adapt to a stimulus, or lose fat. Once we have ascertained that goal, we can decide how long we can stay, and to what degree, in one state. This will consider what we metabolically and hormonally know about the individual.

For example, someone with a genetic disposition to a higher level of androgens and GH the "athletic" type may be able to stay in a destructive metabolism for longer periods without the inevitable "cost" to muscle tissue being too high. They can lose fat faster while preserving muscle better (due largely to better protein synthesis). This is why we must always consider the individual with any strategy we implement and consider that strategy's pros and cons.

Once caloric intake is ascertained and the goal determined, fluctuations between states can be relatively well managed. This also allows us to better understand why simplicity in the early stages of any dietary protocol is highly effective, particularly in obese populations.

Decide where you wish to stay from that point: a surplus, a deficit, or a fluctuation between the two over a given period. Considering my previous point about androgen-dominant individuals, this is why (in general) natural bodybuilders need to diet slower and longer than their assisted counterparts. Fat loss is slower and lean tissue loss will always be greater.

This was also discussed in the research of Helms.[199] There are no absolutes or mathematical formulas with this: only an educated start point followed by some meticulous observation, trial, error, and adjustments.

Once an average caloric level is established, you can then look at this as either a daily target or a longer duration goal. If we base an average off this, giving us a deficit over the course of seven days, we can strategically place higher calorie days when regeneration needs to be prioritized, thus offsetting the negative adaptive metabolic changes. This brings us to the pursuit of building mass while concurrently (remember this term is reflective of time) losing body fat. This notion is not only something I would support through my own observations but one studies have corroborated.

In obese populations, it must be considered that in a caloric deficit of food intake, the abundance of stored energy is not only fuel (if required) but will contribute to weight and fat loss when used. Although it is not identified, it could be suggested that the higher degree of stored fuel (body fat and glycogen) someone may have, the more likely this outcome is.[182–189]

Davoodi et al.[185] performed a study using a calorie-shifted diet (CSD) with a group of overweight women. Calorie shifting is a term synonymous with refeeding. It notes the placement of a caloric or nutrient excess in response to a period in which that marker has been lowered.

Although there are limited studies looking at such protocols, the use of refeeding within bodybuilding preparation has been used with notable success for a considerable time. Davoodi et al. looked at 74 subjects (body mass index ≥25; 37) all of whom were randomized to a four-week control diet, six-week CSD or alternatively CR diets, and a four-week follow-up period.[185]

The study design called for three phases, each two weeks long. Participants would consume 11 days of a CR diet made up of four meals a day separated by four hours without food. This would then be switched to three days ad libitum.

- Phase one 11 days at 1200 k/cal daily, three-day self-regulated refeed
- Phase two 11 days at 1200 k/cal daily, three-day self-regulated refeed
- Phase three 11 days at 1500 k/cal daily, three-self-regulated refeed

The purpose of the caloric increase is to firmly maintain the resting metabolic rate (RMR) to offset any negative adaptations to a prolonged restrictive caloric intake. Again, as in this particular study, we are talking about caloric as opposed substrate intake. On the ad libitum days, there is no noted increase in protein, fats, or carbohydrates beyond the 20:25:50% ratio they controlled on the regulated days.

I would say it would be naive to think they would refeed on higher ratios of proteins and fats, but we cannot rule it out. Under the assumption it was a higher ratio of carbohydrates (as most people would resonate toward), we can make the following metabolic assumptions based on the consequence of refeed days:[168,186–195]

- There would be elevation in thyroid output.
- It would help regulate hunger through altering both leptin and ghrelin levels positively (satiety hormones).

- There would be a decrease in the catecholamine effect and a lowering of cortisol.
- There would be an increase in total and free testosterone.

Obviously, this is still indicative of total caloric intake over a given time.
The up-regulation of metabolism is limited. Caloric intake that is too high will increase body fat.[196]

On ad libitum days, in which full freedom was given, there will be certain individuals for which such a strategy may not be feasible, as they cannot be left "uncontrolled" or with loose rules to follow. Food relationships, behaviors, metabolic state, etc. must all be considered.

SUBSTRATES

Part of the process of nutrient cycling or the manipulation of macronutrients is to allow more metabolic flexibility the body's ability to switch between insulin- and glucagon-mediated pathways.

After establishing a caloric base point, the next goal is to place different demands on these differing physiological states. To establish the desired caloric levels, we need to vary the levels of carbohydrates and dietary fats because each is predominantly determined by glucose and lipid oxidation.

This is where finding someone's "sweet spot" of carbohydrate intake may take some time; it will require trial and error and other considerations discussed later in this chapter. A slight abundance of amino acids made available for fuel serve to protect lean mass when in a hypocaloric state. The chronic absence of carbs also plays its role in this. This is why, for many, low-carb dieting yields diminishing returns over time.

People with more body fat to lose would typically resonate toward a higher amount of time in lipid oxidation; therefore, carbohydrates would be lower on average. As they get leaner, this number would concomitantly increase. Again, this will increase as an average of overall intake until that sweet spot is found.

Too many people stay in the low-carb regimen way too long. Often, people consider carbs in the following way: carbs lowered = weight loss; carbs increased = weight gain. This is part of the reason people feel carbs should be excluded from their diet.

As a coach, it is imperative to explain why carbs are necessary, how to reintroduce them, and how to include them throughout. This brings us to carb cycling, which is a relatively simple wave-pattern concept. Carb cycling allows us to stimulate a higher level of lipid oxidation while fueling and protecting tissue through the glucose-mediated pathways. The elevation of dietary fats also serves to support various other metabolically important systems.

There are dozens of variations on the structure of carb cycling, but generally, they rotate around a three-day cycle nearly exclusively used with those needing finer changes to composition. All three carb days would be reflected with either moderated or a slightly lower fat and protein intake.

The protein intake would generally remain more consistent. Should caloric intake vary, the fats and carbs would help maintain regulation. Establish a carb intake reflective of goals and current intake (ideally an established "sweet spot").

The low-carb day may see the continued regulation of even higher protein and higher fats, should caloric levels require it. These may even be "no" carb days in some cases. By default, protein is only moved due to the lower carb days. This, in many protocols, is kept consistent with the only two actual variables being carbs and perhaps fats. In restrictive caloric states, data is pointing us in the region of 2.3–3 g/kg of bodyweight of protein. In equilibrium or hypercaloric states, this number would perhaps be slightly less.

The manipulation of nutrients is fine and certainly has its place. But remember, the more complex something is, the less consistent it can be. For many, compliance is a bigger fish to fry. Once compliance is achieved, more advanced manipulations become useful and, in some cases, necessary. Humans naturally do this anyways. In many cases, people have been nutrient cycling for many years tracking nutrients and making specific and result-oriented manipulations.

PROTEIN INTAKE

> *"Everything we do, everything we are, and everything we become depends on the action of thousands of different proteins"*
> *~Houston*[197]

In any program intent on physical adaptation or change, protein intake is one of the most critical elements. Much like the necessity to influence meal frequency is still somewhat equivocal, science gives us suggestive markers, which would lead to us minimizing the risk of the body digging into its own amino acid pool as opposed to those obtained from diet.

If adaptation or physiological change is our goal, the need for adequate protein in energy surplus, balance, and deficit is critical in maintaining or increasing lean mass. In surplus or balance, the demand on amino acids as a fuel source is reduced due to the adequate supply of alternative substrates in particular carbohydrates. Carbs act in a protein-sparing capacity, thus allowing amino acids to be used for repair and adaptation as opposed to an alternative source of energy.

This is significant when we consider a deficit is required for fat loss or catabolic processes and a surplus is required for anabolic processes. The level of dietary protein and its influence on whole-body protein utilization is critical in this balance. Remember, protein turnover = protein synthesis/protein breakdown.

One the main priorities is to minimize uncontrolled protein breakdown (proteolysis) and maximize protein synthesis. This, as previously mentioned, is partly the purpose behind minimizing both emotional and physical stressors. Cascades such as cortisol dysregulation affect thyroid hormone levels, leading to the reduction in protein breakdown all of which play a role. This is also why the chronic abstinence of carbs over time becomes detrimental to muscle mass.

In the pursuit of physical adaptation, we must prioritize our training toward our ultimate goals. Despite the debate between the efficacy of different training modalities on anabolic and catabolic processes, it is apparent nutrition plays a large role. Further, changes in nutrition can be used to offset any excessive regression from one's goals. With the right nutritional practices, almost any exercise pursuit can be enjoyed without overly compromising physical goals in the general populous. Remember that a large amount of the research we collate is based on finicky minute details and people end up worrying or blaming indiscriminate things for a lack of physical progress.

> *"Without using some cliché quote about the necessity for exercise to be fun, the compliance of someone with anything must come with some level of enjoyment be it before, during, after, or as a by-product of the activity. Many people never experience how it feels to be truly content in their skin. They can, therefore, never understand something they've never experienced. It is like looking at a rollercoaster and saying, "What kind of fool would go on that?"'*
> *~Phil Learney*

However, it is also apparent that many "exercise" pursuits are done less often merely for enjoyment, but with the belief that it is a pathway to a specific goal (usually fat loss). Fat loss is about nutrition and energy usage it is not much more complicated than that. Therefore, we need a system with efficient energy pathways, yet paradoxically, at the point of usage, equally inefficient systems.

Now let's consider protein intake and where it needs to be. In chapter 8, we discussed meal frequency, specifically how it attempts to maintain an adequate amino acid pool. It makes sense that whatever the chosen meal frequency, the best scenario is to evenly split intake over those meals. If you fail to hit the target number of meals one day, do not stress at the inordinate amount of size or gains you may lose.
Chronic and repeated mistakes are all that should concern us and these can be

bracketed under the "habit" umbrella and one that would be negative long term. Avoid mistakes through planning and understanding your terrain. If it happens as this is life and often it gets in the way of itself do not fret. Do what you can to rectify it and move on. Do not worry about a mistake. In all honesty, missing a meal will not do most people as much harm as the guilt trip they send themselves on for the rest of the day.

There is an enormous amount of data out there regarding protein. The only real certainty we have is that the 0.8 g/kg recommended daily allowance probably needs some updating, as it is largely based on structural requirements and the prevention of deficiency as opposed to rectifying an excess of breakdown. This figure is also based largely on the hypothesis that tissue maintenance revolves around the nitrogen balance within the body. The methodology used in measuring the nitrogen balance is not a tissue-specific measurement; therefore, it cannot truly be seen as an accurate measure when considering tissue loss or gain.

During the breakdown of amino acids, we must consider the capacity of the liver to delaminate them. During this process, the amount of urea in the body will naturally elevate. Often, it will be seen in the blood tests of those with higher-protein diets. This is because there is a maximal rate of urea excretion that can be achieved by the body.[198]

As a rule, elevation of protein intake does not alter this. Therefore, the rate of dietary protein breakdown by the liver and according elevation in urea is determined by individual factors. These factors include bodyweight and the amount of protein used for tissue growth, hormone production, etc. (not required to be delaminated) outlined by the recommended daily allowance. Increased addition of protein under the various dietary circumstances discussed would add to the body's energy need through gluconeogenesis or as stored fat. The "weight loss" advantage of high-protein diets shown in some studies is partly due to its higher rate of thermogenesis and its actions on satiety.

Rudman et al.[198] developed an algorithm to estimate the maximal rate of urea synthesis (MRUS) that gives us theoretical levels of consumption before symptoms of hyperammonemia and hyperaminoacidemia become evident.

The literature seems to support that athletic populations and those seeking muscular adaptation should be looking at a baseline of 1.2–2.2 g/kg. More recent literature from Helms et al.[199] stated that protein needs for energy-restricted resistance-trained athletes are likely 2.3–3.1 g/kg of FFM, scaled upwards with severity of caloric restriction and leanness.

When looking at this, we must also consider the level of protein breakdown across specific activities. We can top the breakdown tree with bodybuilding because its overall intent is the increase in breakdown through training alongside the increase in synthesis through dietary intake. In some cases, this is joined with the use of drug assistance. What we clearly know is that an increase in dietary protein positively impacts nitrogen retention, leucine oxidation, and the rate of protein turnover.[200–204]

The conclusions of Helms et al.[199] would suggest that the steeper the level of caloric restriction and the leaner the athlete, the more the supportive requirements of protein are needed. More recent studies have pointed at much higher levels of intake being effective. But again, in many, the consideration of the activity, the protein-sparing impact of other nutrients, caloric intake, protein source, etc. all appear quite liberal.

If we consider the preceding factors, the balance between digestible protein and actual energy intake must be considered to spare protein. There is some interesting data with respect to protein-sparing modified-fast diets, but almost all of the data is gathered around overweight or obese individuals.

There are several arguments here. First, that due to the level of adiposity gained over a long duration, the alterations in the HTPA axis and the various metabolic adaptations would indicate that, despite a level of lean tissue loss, the baseline level of muscle protein would have been spared as a matter solely of the function of bodyweight versus movement. Second, at the other end of the scale, with lean individuals, the lack of subcutaneous fat would lend a higher ratio of amino acids to be broken down in a caloric deficit just as means of survival.[199,205,206]

Note that as obesity levels rise, there is an inherent surplus of fuel reserves. In most cases, the surplus of fuel reserves concurrently rises with various metabolic adaptations and dysfunctions. In a perfect scenario, extremes of hypocaloric dieting could, in theory, be sustained when these fuel reserves are high (heightened levels of body fat). The need for more accurate caloric control to manage composition would therefore become more apparent as body fat levels decrease.

You could argue that with elevated degrees of obesity, a hypocaloric diet does not necessarily mean that the body is in a fuel deficit in fact, it has an abundance of reserves.

Depending on the degree of obesity, caloric control is initially more about compliance and positively adjusting the behaviors surrounding food. Lean mass due to TBM may well be protected as a simple method of physiological movement and mechanical requirements. The need for complex methods to initiate fat loss is unnecessary and a simple control of dietary intake (k/cal) with an increase in output would lend itself to a higher ratio of fat loss.

People with higher degrees of body fat will use up a higher ratio of FM:FFM than their lean counterparts. The inherent decline in protective androgens that occurs with dieting opens them up further to usage as fuel. This is perhaps one of the reasons many natural physique athletes that diet yearly for competitions fail to notably improve on overall mass. The diets are too short and therefore too extreme. It would then be advisable under periods of caloric restriction to get a higher ratio of your caloric intake from protein sources.[205,206]

Studies have shown that under periods of caloric restriction, muscle tissue is susceptible to loss and the leaner an individual, the higher this ratio is. An incremental increase in protein relevant to the caloric deficit would be advisable in almost all cases.[134,136,199,205,208–211]

It has also been shown that any kind of testosterone therapy enhances muscle mass due to an increase in muscle protein synthesis. This would suggest that the higher an individual's natural or pharmacologically assisted androgen level may be, the greater the protein synthesis and imposed demand for the substrate.[212]

When striving for maximal protein synthesis (MPS), we must also consider several other factors. Leucine is a major factor in protein synthesis and the ability of dietary proteins to be of use in tissue regeneration. Leucine levels at 0.05 g/kg have been shown to saturate the mammalian target of rapamycin (mTOR) pathways, increasing MPS.[213]

In summary, it could be suggested that any individual undertaking any type of athletic endeavor should use a protein intake between 1.2–2.2 g/kg, under the assumption that basal caloric requirements are met or exceeded. Most of this data is based on TBM, not LBM.

Protein intake would significantly increase in a caloric deficit and with a decreased level of adiposity. In many cases, this would supersede basal recommendations. It is suggested this would be between 2.3-3.1 g/kg of LBM in restrictive circumstances.[208]

Drug-assisted bodybuilders using androgens would further increase muscle protein synthesis. Despite a lack of research, it could be hypothesized that muscle protein synthesis could be as high as 2.9 g–3.9 g/kg of LBM. There could also be further consideration for those using thyroid drugs, beta agonists, and peptides.[212] Non-drug-assisted bodybuilders would therefore serve better with longer, less aggressive diets to minimize destructive metabolism. This would also remain true for any fat loss approach.

CARBOHYDRATES

Carbohydrates are probably the most hotly debated of the macronutrients. The main role of carbohydrates within the body is to provide cellular fuel and to help facilitate the metabolism of fat. Carbohydrates yield 4 k/cal of energy per gram.[214] Let's look at carbohydrates, beginning with their structure. There are four major types of carbohydrates: polysaccharides, monosaccharides, disaccharides, and oligosaccharides. These are commonly referred to as complex carbohydrates, formed primarily of starches and fibers (polysaccharides) and simple sugars made up of a single molecule (monosaccharides, the most common being glucose, fructose, and galactose). Disaccharides contain two molecules and oligosaccharides contain between two and ten molecules. The more complex polysaccharides form a very large molecule made up of hundreds or thousands of molecules.

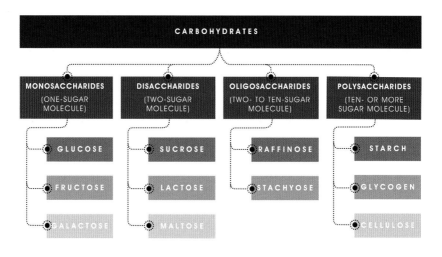

Figure 12 Illustration of carbohydrates and their chemical compositions.

These classifications of carbohydrates help us understand their transference, passage, and absorption from ingestion to a usable cellular fuel. The speed at which it travels from the small intestine to the blood will dictate its most effective use within a dietary regimen.

For us to make use of any form of carbohydrate as a cellular fuel source, it must first be digested and then hydrolyzed into monosaccharides. Upon ingestion of different types of foodstuffs, the body produces enzymes to act as catalysts in the breakdown of complex structures in to their simpler usable formats. In the case of carbohydrates, the ones most of note are those of starches or polysaccharides. Irrespective of the type, if the body is deficient in a saccharide, it can create any type from glucose through various enzymatic and molecular steps.

After (and, to some degree, before) the ingestion of starches, the salivary glands, pancreas, and small intestine produce amylase, the enzymatic catalyst that allows the breakdown of these more complex forms. In this digestible starch, the enzymes are unable to break down the bonds of what we term "resistant starch," but are most commonly referred to as dietary fiber.

Once digested, monosaccharides are absorbed into the bloodstream through the small intestine. This is when we start to get into the topic of the glycemic index (GI): the ranking of food based on its blood glucose response. Various carbohydrates will conform to a high and rapid response or a slower and low response and the range between.

The higher the rise in glucose, the more insulin should be produced in response by the beta cells of the pancreas; this is referred to as the glucose-sensitive insulin secretion (GSIS). Diminished function GSIS is tantamount to buying your weekly shopping but only taking one carrier bag.

The glucose has no carrier (insulin) to transport it to cells, so it remains circulating in the bloodstream. Over time, this state perpetuates the problem and often leads to the various stages of insulin resistance, beta-cell dysfunction, and the issues we associate with type 2 onset diabetes.

In regulating this response, low and medium GI foods are often suggested as a carbohydrate of choice. Alternatively, short-term lowering of total carbohydrate intake to rectify the insulinogenic response and bring up insulin sensitivity is also a suitable strategy. Remember that someone demonstrating an impaired glucose tolerance will not be able to release insulin rapidly to coincide with a rapid rise in blood glucose.

The concentration of glucose in the blood is the main regulator of insulin secretion by the pancreas. If this level of glucose increases rapidly or remains high, so does the synthesis of insulin. If the level of glucose is low, the level of insulin drops concurrently with a rise in glucagon. The normal concentration of glucose in plasma is 5 mmol/l and any level above this will cause an increase in the secretory rate of insulin and therefore a decrease in glucagon.

The body is in a regulatory pattern; therefore, the level of glucose in plasma tends to stay relatively constant under healthy circumstances, with the level of insulin circulating being the larger variant of the two. Insulin is one of the key controllers of this set point, alongside the regulatory and counter-regulatory neurohormonal system.

Any variability brought about by adverse dietary patterns and what appear to be chronically high blood glucose levels above ~11 mmol/l have implications with diabetes mellitus, insulin resistance, and beta-cell dysfunction. Other fluxes are brought about by alterations in uptake, retention, and disposal rates. But, as a general rule, if there is an increase in exit rates, there is simultaneously an increase in delivery to stabilize levels.[215]

During any prolonged period of carbohydrate restriction, a decrease in plasma glucose as little as 20 mg/dl (from 90–70 mg/dl) causes a decrease in glucose metabolism and thus signals the onset of hypoglycemia and the release of the counter-regulatory hormones glucagon, catecholamines, cortisol, and GH.[216]

This supports a shift from insulin-mediated energy pathways to glucagon-mediated pathways.[217–218] The switch between these pathways may cause short-term issues for many. Ways in which we may temporarily offset this will be discussed in the next section when considering fats, but it is largely due to a simple transient adaptation period.

Within the typical Western diet, the average person consumes about 300 g of carbohydrates daily.[219] Consider that a healthy functioning adult can store approximately 400 g as muscle glycogen, 90–110 g as liver glycogen, and 25 g circulates in the blood as glucose.[220] Under normal conditions, the skeletal muscle glycogen concentration is between 1.5–2 g/100 g skeletal muscle.[221-224] Fluctuating blood glucose, poor insulin secretion, cellular resistance, and overindulgent dietary practices all play a part in an excess of carbohydrates being consumed, given the individual's physiological circumstances.

Now, if we move the body out of normal conditions and look to deplete glycogen stores the body is able to increase storage capacity by over 50%. It should be noted, however, that most of these studies were completed with endurance athletes: the capacity of weight-trained athletes may potentially exceed this.

CARBOHYDRATES AND WEIGHT LOSS

The vast majority of weight loss most will see from low-carb diets is brought about by the alteration in cellular fluid levels and calorie reduction. Remember that any "weight loss" strategy usually revolves around a common food type or group someone removes, not replaces, thus lowering the net amount of calories consumed. Telling the average Westerner to omit carbohydrates, gluten, or another nutrient from their diet is not typically treated as replacement advice. The individual merely lowers net caloric intake by omitting something from their diet that previously played a large role in their intake.

This helps us understand the methods that periodically and intentionally deplete levels of glycogen, particularly in weight/fat loss regimens. It also outlines the necessity not to exclude carbohydrates for any chronic period. The period of time in which cells may uptake these aforementioned amounts will depend on various factors, including the degree of beta-cell function, glucose disposal, and total LBM. If we correlate this with obesity, it suggests the total amount of carbs would be lower and cellular refeeds would need to be longer in more obese populations. In addition, the management of carbohydrates with a smaller molecular number of saccharides and higher GI may well be poorly managed in such populations. The inclusion of more complex, fibrous, and lower glycemic carbs may yield better benefits in the early stages of weight loss.

Looking to the Future of Workout Carbohydrates

Cyclodextrins (cycloamyloses) are produced from starch using enzymatic conversion. They are largely manufactured for use by the pharmaceutical companies as a method of drug delivery that does not induce spikes or fast release into the bloodstream. This has led the sport supplement industry to look at starches differently. Substances with a high molecular weight and low osmolality (how much water is drawn around a molecule) will rapidly pass through the gastric system, allowing a faster absorption of critical nutrients.

This has prompted their development for use in pre-, intra- and post-workout nutrition. One of most note is highly branched cyclic dextrin (HBCD). HBCD is broken down using amylopectin that, alongside glycogen, is a highly branched polymer found in plants and is a soluble polysaccharide. Fundamentally, the more branches a compound has, the more end points enzymes can be attached to; therefore, it can be degraded or hydrolyzed faster.

Readily taking in carbohydrates as we workout serves multiple purposes. It allows us to keep blood glucose at a steady state, fueling the working muscles and enabling a higher work capacity (assuming it gets there fast enough to do so). It also allows the highly anabolic hormone, insulin, to come into play. Insulin will help protein synthesis, ensuring that the catabolic actions of protein breakdown are kept to a minimum.

So why is HBCD superior to dextrose or other simple carbohydrates? Once carbohydrates are transported into the stomach, they are broken down into smaller chains of glucose and maltose (two glucose molecules) that are then absorbed by the small intestine.

However, we must first consider the stage before these molecules move into the small intestine. Both the molecular weight and osmolality of the molecule will factor into how quickly the gastric emptying will be, which is the rate of transport into the small intestine.

The small intestine has a series of receptors called osmoreceptors that detect the osmolality of the molecule as it exits the stomach. If the molecule has a high osmolality, gastric emptying rates will be slowed. The fact that dextrose and simple carbs are often referred to as "fast" carbs is just an indicator of capacity.

This is tantamount to having two racecars: one with a 9000-rpm capacity and the other with a 1000-rpm capacity. The 9000-rpm capacity car also has a time-release clutch, meaning it can be incredibly fast, but it takes time for the clutch to be fully released. The 1000-rpm capacity car has a regular clutch and the clutch is fully released right away.

In this analogy, the "clutch" is the rate of passage into the small intestine. In the "slow" car, the adsorption is steady, keeping blood glucose and the demand on insulin as a carrier steady as well. In the "fast" car, the adsorption from the small intestine to the bloodstream is rapid. Once the clutch is dropped, blood sugar increase and insulin spikes. This creates the environment we want. However, the adsorption rate, coupled with the GI of the carb, can drive the body into hyperglycemia, which is often rapidly followed by an accompanying drop into hypoglycemia.

This is more of a concern in today's society because many people have compromised beta-cell function, their GSIS is not what it used to be, and cell receptors can be damaged. Further, the delay in emptying and level of water drawn around the molecule causes a level of gastric distress, which is exacerbated by a workout.

There are many advancements in polymers and "carrying" compounds, but these again are reserved for the pre-, intra-, and post-workout period, when they become of functional use.

FATS

Dietary fats, the most calorically dense of the macronutrients, yield nine calories per gram, as opposed to the four calories both protein and carbohydrates yield. Dietary fats earned a bad reputation due to their caloric density and the respective lack of food volume. Thus, upon removal from any dietary regimen, the resultant loss in weight was always attributed to the macronutrient itself as opposed to the larger drop in overall calories.

If we consider generational trends and, to some degree, fear mongering those who grew up in the 1970s and 1980s will more than likely still have a learned need to avoid fats. Dietary fats are referred to as triglycerides, which are composed of three fatty acids and a molecule of glycerin. Through the process of digestion, lipase (the enzyme that breaks down fats) is released by the pancreas. Lipids are hydrophobic; therefore, the way they are handled in cells differs greatly from other molecules involved in metabolism.

Almost all lipids are classed as non-polar and (in contrast to those classified as polar) do not have a degree of electrical charge, which allows them to mix and combine with water. Sugar and salt are hydrophilic, meaning they mix with water; hence, the cellular drawing actions of both these substances. This, combined with molecular size and polarity, will influence the substances' cell permeability.
The main roles of fatty acids are to provide the structural integrity of cell

membranes, act as a raw material for conversion into other substances, and serve as an energy source.

Due to the fats being hydrophobic, the lipase that is released cannot act on them. To achieve this, bile is secreted from the liver and gallbladder, emulsifying the fat into smaller parts and therefore more surface area for the enzyme to act upon. Bile is amphipathic, which means it is a molecule with both polar and non-polar aspects. The bile forms a bridge between the polar and non-polar regions, allowing the fats to break down and lipase to do its job.

Once the fats are emulsified, they form small droplets that allow lipase to act upon them and pass through the bloodstream. Both mechanisms are critical; therefore, we once again underline the importance of liver and pancreatic health in metabolic function.

Due to this breakdown, fats do not require a carrier they simply permeate cells once broken down into their raw components. After lipase and bile act upon them, dietary fats are broken down into fatty acids and glycerol. Fatty acids provide fuel and act on metabolic functions, whereas glycerol can be used as glucose.

Fatty acids are categorized in many ways; the fatty acids carbon chain length and type of saturation dictate many characteristics, including their melting point. The longer the chain is, the higher the fat melting point. Fats are then categorized by their degree of saturation: either saturated or unsaturated. Finally, by the location of their double bonds, it is determined whether they are omega-3 or omega-6 fatty acids.

The length of carbon chain categorizes fats as:

- Short-chain fatty acids less than six carbons; sources: butyric acid, caproic acid
- Medium-chain fatty acids six to twelve carbons; sources: lauric acid, myristic acid, and caprylic acid
- Long-chain fatty acids twelve or more carbons; sources: palmitic acid, stearic acid, and arachidic acid

Fats cannot be used during high-intensity exercise as fuel, so the notion that high-intensity exercise burns fat is a myth. Lipids are only used in aerobic metabolism and not anaerobic processes. However, high-intensity exercise can mobilize fatty acids to be concurrently used for energy as intensity lowers or between high-intensity bouts. It is an indirect process.

TYPES OF DIETARY FATS

There are three basic types of fatty acid: saturated, polyunsaturated, and monounsaturated. Saturated fats are still the brunt of many medical myths and a somewhat unwarranted association with and correlation to heart disease. This has been debunked notably over the past few years, with the focus being placed upon the type and subtypes of cholesterol. However, knowledge still seems to be lagging behind the science.[225–227]

LDL, the protein that carries cholesterol through the blood, has always been linked with heart disease and broadly labeled as the "bad" cholesterol. We are now however aware of two subtypes of LDL and only one is of major concern. The two subtypes are categorized by their size and ability to pass through arterial walls. Small, dense LDL is of most concern, whereas the larger LDL is unable to pass through walls; therefore, the elevation of blood cholesterol becomes negligible. It must be noted that saturated fats also raise the "good" cholesterol (HDL).[228–230]

The basic structure of saturated fats would generally mean that, at room temperature, they are solid and have a longer life. Unsaturated fats, however, have a different chemical structure that leaves them open to going rancid. The term "saturated" comes from the fact that they are saturated with hydrogen atoms.

Each carbon molecule only has space for two hydrogen atoms and they are all full. In the case of unsaturated or the mono- and polyunsaturated fats, a double bond forms in the space left by hydrogen atoms. The fats we consume are a ratio of all three types.

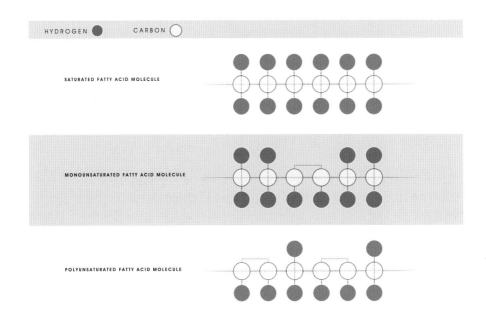

Figure 13 Illustration of the chemical structure of various types of fatty acids.

If observed under microscopic conditions, there would be a bend in the molecule at the double bond. This is what makes unsaturated fats liquid, as opposed to the straight chain solid form of saturated fats. It also makes them volatile and likely to become rancid. This is overcome in food manufacture through hydrogenation. As the name implies, it means the fats are treated with hydrogen to increase shelf life. The by-product of this is trans fats or trans fatty acids, as they are also known.

The restriction of dietary fats in someone's diet <20% total intake, would, over time, lead to a lowering of:

- Mineralocorticoids Responsible for sodium, potassium, water, and mineral metabolism alongside the actions of the kidneys.[231]
- Glucocorticoids Responsible for intermediary metabolism, inflammation, immunity, wound healing, and myocardial and muscular integrity. They are also largely responsible in stimulating the conversion of protein to carbohydrates in gluconeogenesis. The need for fats when moving down glucagon-based metabolic pathways is critical.[232]
- Androgens Androgens are the group of sex hormones often categorized as "male" hormones due to their impact on male morphological development. However, androgens are crucial for both male and female sexual and reproductive function alongside their secondary sexual characteristics such as body and facial hair and bone and muscular development. Androgens can also inhibit the ability of some fats to store lipids.[233–239]

- Progestogens Progestogens, such as progesterone, help regulate menstruation and gestation hormones. If estrogen levels get too high, progesterone can no longer maintain a dynamic balance. Progesterone assists in the formation of new bone, regulation of blood pressure, fat storage, and carbohydrate metabolism.
- Vitamin D Technically a secosteroid (or hormone precursor) but functions as a steroidal hormone. Converted in the liver, it serves many metabolic and supportive functions.

The general recommendations for dietary fat suggest between 20–30% of total caloric intake should come from fats. In athletic populations, this number seems to range between 30–50%.[240]

Insulin, catecholamines, and various other hormones are responsible for the breakdown of fats into glycerol and fatty acids (lipolysis). Three enzymes play a large part in this breakdown: adipose triglyceride lipase (ATGL), HSL, and monoacylglycerol lipase (MGL). Triglycerides are present in both adipose tissue and muscle tissue. Once broken down and freed from glycerol, these fatty acids can diffuse into the blood or muscle fibers to be used as fuel.

The inclusion of dietary fats (and at what level) is dictated by the overall energy balance and intent of the dietary regimen. If switching substrates in dietary intake, fats would typically be elevated against a baseline protein amount and a variable carb amount. The higher inclusion of dietary fats would be apparent in varying degrees of metabolic dysfunction, relation differentials, and a potential degree of obesity (remember, this is not a given but a correlation and certain individuals may not have the proposed dysfunction).

There remains an extreme debate between supporters of carbs and supporters of fat. Once again, we are attempting to sit on either side of the proverbial fence. It becomes a battle of extremes, much like the clean versus flexible eating debate. However, the inclusion of all macronutrients within any dietary regimen has its time and place. There seems to be an inherent need to stand in a corner and fight instead of embracing what is great about each nutrient and utilizing those aspects when required.

The mark of a good coach is acknowledging when something be it a method or system is most applicable to that individual given their circumstances. Too many people need absolutes and want someone to come up with the system.

In summary, the main goal is to consider the initial physiological state of the individual and their dietary history and correlate it with their goals. If exercise performance or an increase in lean mass is the goal, as opposed to fat loss, the insulin-mediated pathways will undoubtedly be used more and glycogen stores become critical to more prolonged exercise bouts and higher volume bodybuilding-style workouts. Alongside this, the lipolysis of fats becomes less of a focus, so insulin can remain raised pre-, intra- and post-workout. If glucagon is to be raised to help in the breakdown of fatty acids, the occlusion of carbohydrates prior to a workout would therefore be useful.

Find the sweet spot of intake that manages sustainable energy levels and the goal at hand. Look not only at daily totals, but at the amount over given cycles. As mentioned before, the subtle similarities in training periodization are not that dissimilar to nutrition. This level of tolerance or intake will be related to the individual's total lean mass and their degree of beta-cell function, glucose uptake, and clearance rates (this can also be related to the type of exercise they are undertaking).

We could loosely correlate this with the degree of obesity, but this merely gives us a higher possibility that the aforementioned functions have indeed become compromised. To draw any conclusions based on this fact would be short thinking, but to ignore the likelihood may be unwise.

Over time, with the correct nutritional strategy, carbohydrate tolerance will increase alongside compositional status. The ultimate goal, once again, is the ability to switch between different pathways easily and to facilitate energy from any of the three macronutrients, should there be a demand to do so. In conjunction with this, a degree of flexibility in dietary choices may not exist right now, given the metabolically compromising problems.

Chapter 13: Metabolic Hormones

We are currently seeing cases in which, over time, the cells, glands, and receptors in the body are becoming overwhelmed and, in many cases, resistant to the specific hormonal actions that regulate them. These then become compromised, both creating and supporting the cascade of negative physiological and psychological changes that can occur.

To create a better understanding of these happenings, basic knowledge of certain hormones associated with metabolic function and protein synthesis would be useful. Insulin, glucagon, the aforementioned catecholamines (adrenaline and noradrenaline), the thyroid hormones, the satiety hormones (leptin and ghrelin), and testosterone (of the androgens) remain most noteworthy.

To understand metabolic hormones, we must first understand the fundamentals of hormones and their actions. The primary role of hormones is to communicate between the cells within the body.

The hypothalamus acts as both the regulator and link for hormones between the central nervous system (CNS) and the remainder of tissue mediated by homeostatic signals. In response to these homeostatic signals, neural signals are converted into hormonal responses.

Circadian rhythm alters hypothalamic hormone release according to a 24-hour cycle. This alters metabolic rate, digestion, body temperature, and blood pressure accordingly. These alterations should be considered alongside adjustments in other ever-changing aspects such as emotional and physical stressors, hydration, or blood pressure. The term we use for these primary stage hormones are "releasing" hormones.

INSULIN

Insulin, if we talk about in a simplified manner, is a hormone secreted to regulate blood glucose levels or after the consumption of food. Glucose (carbs and sugars) is its main mediator, but all foods have an insulinogenic effect that would also become dependent upon other factors within the individual's diet.

Using a more in-depth explanation: glucose transporter type two (GLUT-2) mediates the entry of glucose into beta cells. This is the raw fuel for glycolysis, our standard energy-producing pathway; glucose is phosphorylated by the rate-limiting enzyme glucokinase. Often referred to as the master hormone, insulin plays a large regulatory role.

Further, it has earned a somewhat unjust bad reputation, largely due to the misunderstanding surrounding its inhibitory actions. Insulin inhibits lipolysis (breakdown of fats) with phosphatidylinositol 3-kinase (PI3K) and phosphodiesterase 3 (PDE3), stimulating the re-esterification of FFAs. This results in an inhibition of FFA release (mobilization of fats to be used as fuel).[241,242] This, however, serves to protect all stored metabolites, including amino acids, and therefore assists in the preservation of lean mass.

As lean tissue is critical for most compositional improvements, both insulin production and carbohydrate intake are critical for a multitude of reasons.

After the consumption of any meal, we produce an elevated rise in insulin secretion, which can either be glucose-mediated (GSIS) or non-glucose-mediated, so formed through the insulinemic properties of fats and proteins or by the incretins glucose-dependent insulinotropic peptide (GIP) and glucagon-like peptide-1 (GLP-1), which are a group of gastrointestinal hormones that react to the glucose concentrations in the lumen of the digestive tract.

This stimulation of counter-regulatory hormones initiates a shift away from carbohydrate metabolism through acknowledgment of a variability of insulin concentrations. This signals the release of glucagon by the alpha cells of the pancreas, thus switching to the metabolic use of amino and/or fatty acids. This is what we refer to as gluconeogenesis.

Once glucose actually enters the bloodstream via absorption through the intestine, breakdown of liver glycogen or from gluconeogenesis in the actual liver initiates a secretion of insulin. Insulin binds to receptors in the liver, kidneys, muscle, and adipose tissue once this rise in glucose concentration is detected. This then inhibits the liver and kidneys from releasing any further glucose that would be required to maintain this level of plasma glucose in the absence of dietary influence.

Insulin secretion occurs in two phases. The first is initiated when the pancreas detects a rise in glucose. The pancreas responds by releasing stored insulin and ceases within 10 minutes, which is further enhanced by the incretin hormones. This first phase serves to reduce basal glucagon secretion and therefore reduces hepatic glucose production. The greater the level of insulin resistance or indeed beta-cell dysfunction, the more this rapid release will be impaired and compromised.

If glucose then remains elevated beyond this point, it moves into what we class as second-phase release. Second-phase release is sustained by beta cells, creating new insulin through synthesis of pre-proinsulin in the ribosomes of the rough endoplasmic reticulum. This is then broken down into proinsulin, transported to the Golgi apparatus, and broken down once again into equimolar (equal amount of moles) amounts of insulin and c-peptide. This occurs until a stable blood glucose level is established (71–99 mg/dL).[243]

Due to the cleaving process and the two equimolar amounts of insulin and c-peptide, the c-peptide:glucose ratio can be useful as an indicator for beta-cell activity. Put to great use in the treatment of diabetes, it is also a good indicator of the stages leading up to the condition.

The elevation in blood glucose seen during stages of beta-cell regression is not due to the lack of cellular uptake as previously hypothesized and the glucose essentially being "bounced" back into the bloodstream. It is due, in large part, to the inhibitory actions of insulin on the liver being muted.[244]

Under conditions when insulin and blood glucose are low, the liver will establish a baseline of blood sugar by releasing glucose. Through the metabolic processes of gluconeogenesis and glycogenolysis, the body due to the muted inhibition of insulin uncontrollably releases glucose from the liver. In the case of a type 1 diabetic, if hyperglycemia reaches critical levels, ketoacidosis (the production of ketones from the liver) simultaneously occurs. Without external administration of insulin, this can ultimately result in death.

The pancreas, alongside its beta cells, is responsible for insulin secretion. Over time, if this system is overused (for example, through excessive consumption of foods carbs in particular), it becomes overstimulated, down-regulated, and ultimately dysfunctional alongside the receptors that allow the carrier and substrate into the cells. It is a balancing act; we must stimulate without overstimulating as much as we must focus on consumption.

Five endocrine subsets of cells secrete hormones directly into the bloodstream from the pancreas:

- Alpha cells, which produce glucagon
- Beta cells, which produce insulin and amylin
- Delta cells, which produce somatostatin
- Gamma cells, which produce pancreatic polypeptide
- Epsilon cells, which produce ghrelin

GLUCOSE MEDIATION

If we use a ratio of 1:10 for GSIS (which is a reasonable average across diabetic populations), this means that for every 10 g of carbs we consume, the body will use 1 unit of insulin to manage them and act as a substrate carrier into cellular tissue in its converted form, glycogen.

Under fully functional circumstances, the average human produces 24 units of insulin daily at a basal level. Each meal will typically induce a further five to six units to be produced. This would mean an average Westerner consuming three meals a day with a fully functional GSIS would produce 42 units maximum (or fundamentally, if norms are to be accepted, the ability to take 420 g of glycogen into cells). If you do the math at this stage, you will realize why frequency of meals can play a role when attempting to build more lean tissue and capitalize on the benefits of insulin. You can also see the benefit in an increased meal frequency to insulin-resistant populations.

A high percentage of the Western population is in a state of diminished GSIS, obesity, insulin resistance, and en route to eventual type 2 diabetes. Type 2 diabetes is characterized at stage 4 of beta-cell dysfunction. Most of our clientele looking at weight loss will more than likely be at some diminished stage and, uncommonly, at a state of efficient GSIS. This may be speculative, but the demographic we deal with and reach out to will usually be within these parameters. If you doubt the statistics, start getting blood tests done on your clientele. You will soon believe the mess we are in.

In the process of reaching this level of dysfunction, the cells that generally uptake the glycogen via insulin develop insulin resistance. It is like trying to get into nightclubs with limited capacity and dress codes. There are two hundred people (glucose) waiting outside in incorrect attire. There are two different nightclubs: "muscle," which has a large capacity and "liver," which has a slightly smaller capacity and is slightly harder to get into. A van (pancreas) delivers two hundred suits (insulin) appropriate for the dress code. The properly attired people (glucose and insulin) then proceed to the doors of the clubs. If the clubs are full (glycogen saturated), no one is allowed in and they are left to linger outside until someone leaves (glycogen depletion). Otherwise, they go to another nightclub: "fat," which has an unlimited capacity, is easy to get into, and no doormen.

Insulin resistance is when the clubs' capacity goes down due to renovations and people leaving the club very slowly, therefore, making room and letting more people in suits (glucose and insulin) in is hard. Therefore, the doormen (receptors) are more resistant to letting people in. People remain outside (in the blood) with their suits on. The van (pancreas) that delivers the suits continues to deliver more (insulin) because it sees people still standing outside. The suits are not needed, so in response, more people in the wrong attire are called in (glucose) to fill the suits. This vicious cycle continues as people remain circulating outside the clubs (in the bloodstream) or until they move to the "fat" nightclub.

More suits (insulin) are delivered and more people (glucose) are invited until there is space made available in the club or people stop being invited (ingestion of glucose or release by the liver). This gives the club a chance to disperse people and make room by finishing the renovations. As the renovations near completion, the capacity of the clubs goes up (cellular sensitivity) and the doormen become less resistant to letting people in. If the club wants to get more people in and stay at capacity, it must extend capacity (build muscle) and remain functioning (lean), respectively.

The cells now cannot take in fuel like they used to. This is brought about initially by a level of insulin resistance, developing first in the liver then moving on to whole-body resistance.

It is suggested that insulin sensitivity in the liver is important for whole-body insulin function. Any low level of inflammation in the body or liver can impair this function and its signaling. This justifies that the quality of food we ingest should be considered a factor as opposed to just a series of caloric- or macronutrient-based targets.

There is compromised fuel for tissue and numerous other consequences that obviously come alongside that. Further, there is a reduction in carb "tolerance" and an inhibition in both performance and tissue adaptation. The reduction in uptake means that the surplus must go somewhere. This is where we start to run into serious problems.

An overweight person who has consumed carbohydrates and has diminished GSIS and cellular uptake (resistance) will now have a rapid rise in blood glucose, as the glucose is unable to be taken into cells. This means it remains in the blood as opposed to in cells. This elevation in blood glucose leads to the pancreas signaling a continuous release of more insulin (hyperinsulinemia) in its attempt to bring blood glucose down.

As there is no space in the compromised cells, this rarely happens (unless activity creates increased insulin sensitivity and uses up some of what is in the cell). The continuous elevation in circulating insulin now through various pathways signals to the hypothalamus that the individual needs to consume more food, particularly carbs, to bring that level of insulin down. This creates a sense of false hunger. If this individual continues to follow this pattern, the switch that first turns off the food and cravings will never flip.

In non-diabetics dependent upon the stage of beta-cell dysfunction after consumption of carbohydrates, the glucose production by the liver will be suppressed but only in those with healthy beta-cell function. The greater the stage of dysfunction and degree of insulin resistance exhibited, the less this production will be suppressed. This causes the resulting increases in blood glucose through both the impaired GLUT-4 stimulation but primarily the overproduction of glucose by the liver.

In type 1 diabetes, the beta cells become non-functional due to being attacked by the immune system. When blood sugar levels begin to rise, the beta cells are unable to respond with an acute responsive secretion of insulin to regulate the metabolism of glucose. In type 2 diabetes, the beta cells simply cannot keep up with the demand placed upon them. The exact mechanisms as to why this happens are unclear and much hypothetical and speculative reasoning is out there but is far from being conclusive at this stage. As the mechanisms of diabetes are not essentially our focus here, it is not critical we understand the reasoning, only that the condition and regression of beta-cell function exists.

In the case of people with insulin resistance or a declining state of beta-cell mass and function, there is a progressive noted elevation in blood glucose. It is estimated that at diagnosis, 50% of beta-cell function has been lost in type 2 diabetics.[245]

Beta-cell impairment therefore lends itself to high blood glucose with an inhibited yet continuous response by insulin and its precursor proinsulin. The burden over time on the pancreas is evident and shows why, without dietary intervention, this impairment inevitably leads to type 2 diabetes.[173] The high insulin levels at this stage, due to glucose clearance becoming a priority, begin to stimulate appetite. Cells unable to receive insulin and glucose cause a chronically high level of both blood glucose and circulating insulin.

The elevation in insulin causes a release in LPL that serves to inhibit the breakdown of fat cells to be used as fuel. Therefore, the higher the levels of circulating insulin are, the more lipolysis becomes inhibited. Simple sugars, excessive calories, poor glucose clearance, and cellular resistance can all be contributing factors to high insulin.

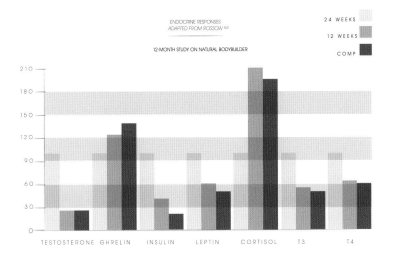

Figure 14 Hormonal and metabolic consequences of contest dieting: adapted from Rossow.[163]

There are six proposed stages of beta-cell dysfunction developed from clinical observation and investigation:[174]

- Stage 0: Normal State Intact acute GSIS.
- Stage 1: Compensation Increased acute GSIS resulting in a higher rate of insulin secretion. A compensated beta-cell mass. Insulin resistance/obesity.
- Stage 2: Stable Adaptation Occurs when glucose levels start to rise and cause disruption of function, as evidenced by a loss of acute GSIS and beta-cell dedifferentiation.
- Stage 3: Unstable Early Compensation A transient unstable period in which glucose levels rise relatively rapidly.
- Stage 4: Stable Decomposition Severe beta-cell dedifferentiation. Type 2 diabetes. Unless rapid autoimmune destruction of the beta cells occurs at this stage, progression to stage 5 would only occur over a long period of time.
- Stage 5: Severe Decompensation A profound reduction in beta-cell mass with progression to ketosis. Type 1 diabetes.

One of the biggest challenges we have here is the ability to clinically gauge the degree of beta-cell mass and function. On a clinical level, one of the most common ways is to test c-peptide. As previously mentioned, during the process of secondary insulin release, insulin and c-peptide are broken off in equal amounts; therefore, this can give us an indication of the amount of insulin being produced. The other of most note is the oral glucose tolerance test (OGTT). Both have their own respective limitations.

As many of us may not have access to lab testing, by understanding of how the OGTT is used, we can utilize various tools and methods of assessment, including simple trial and error.

The first thing we can ascertain about an individual is their current compositional state. This can be done through simple observation or a method previously discussed. In conjunction with a current snapshot of their dietary intake, we can also deduce dietary habits by their responses after periods of food abstinence or their reactions following specific food selections. A historical log at this stage would be advisable.

The OGTT assesses plasma glucose levels in a fasting state. Periodically, following the consumption of a glucose solution, blood is drawn to test glucose levels and, in some cases, insulin. In a fasting state, clinicians are looking for a level below 6.1 mmol/L (110 mg/dL); anything above this, up to 7.0 mmol/L (125 mg/dL), would indicate a degree of beta-cell dysfunction and pre-diabetes. Levels above this range result in a clinical diagnosis of diabetes.

A standard protocol would look at glucose levels 2 hours after consumption: 7.8 mmol/L (140 mg/dL) is the expected level; between 7.8–11.1 mmol/L (140–200 mg/dL) indicates an impaired glucose tolerance; and 11.1 mmol/L (200 mg/dL) or above is the clinical diagnosis for diabetes.

Due to the varying efficiency in people's metabolic processes, you cannot simply conclude there is an inclination toward diabetes due to the level of adiposity. However, in the absence of blood and clinical-level testing, there is simply too much overwhelming evidence to ignore that varying levels of adiposity certainly point toward dysfunction of the insulin-mediated pathways, beta-cell mass, and function and management of carbohydrates in the diet. Remember, tolerance is largely overseen by management. The notion of intolerance appears to be a conclusive state someone will be in; however, with the right intervention, it is leaps and bounds from it.[176]

INTERVENTION

Through the stages of obesity, the degree of insulin resistance will typically rise.[177,246] A major consideration in the dietary prescriptive process is that the closer to stage 5 of beta-cell dysfunction someone becomes, the less efficient they are at processing insulin-mediated glycolysis. Therefore, their required net carbohydrate intake would be lower at that particular stage and there would undoubtedly be a greater reduction in frequency of necessary cellular carbohydrate-oriented "refeeds." The cyclical elevation of calories is of metabolic benefit, but the necessity for carbohydrates to be part of that is less so. Concomitantly, glucose clearance becomes poorer and the "space" in cells for glucose decreases.

As these conditions improve alongside a reduction in fat mass, the frequency and amount of carbohydrates in the diet will therefore increase. Their sensitivity to insulin, their pancreatic efficiency and GSIS, glucose clearance, and control of the appetite center of the brain all improve. It is therefore apparent as to why obese populations appear to have greater success with lower carbohydrate dieting, yet encounter plateaus through long-term continuation of this method.

The potential issues following removal of any substrate from a dietary strategy without any form of educated rationale is potential alienation of that particular nutrient. Furthermore, when you then applaud the client's fat loss around its removal, is it any wonder that people become terrified of certain foods? Much like previous generations still hold a fear of dietary fats, those brought up in the past 20–30 years have that same inherent and unnecessary fear of carbohydrates.

It could be suggested that through increased adiposity, the production of insulin is inhibited. Therefore, active low-level stimulation of insulin through non-glucose-mediated pathways would be beneficial in the early stages of a nutritional strategy.

There appears to be little, if any, stimulation of blood glucose with protein ingestion. However, a relatively low increase in insulin and increased ratio of protein in exchange for the same caloric level of carbohydrates may show an initial benefit, depending on the level of adiposity. Through glucagon-mediated pathways, this would provide cellular glycogen for both working muscle and the liver, while simultaneously minimally increasing blood glucose. Fundamentally, the lowering of carbohydrates would require a relative increase in protein should protection of lean mass be a priority.

Dietary fats would therefore account for the remaining calories. Protein ingested alongside a low ratio of carbohydrates can also improve the postprandial response to carbohydrates. Therefore, long-term management of carbohydrates will improve.[180,181,247–251]

With the implications of such a strategy, it must be noted that the short-term changes in substrate ratios for anyone will create a period of physiological discomfort to some degree. Candidates that would use this type of approach will be carbohydrate-adapted and therefore, in the onset, inefficient in using amino and fatty acids as usable and efficient sources of fuel.

"Studies of elite athletes chronically adapted to low-carbohydrate diets have uncovered one unexpected finding—their extraordinary ability to produce energy at very high rate, purely from the oxidation of fat."

~Noakes et al.[252]

Also, as androidal obesity is associated with increased cortisol secretion, and cortisol secretion initiates gluconeogenesis, the contribution to abnormal glucose metabolism would point us away from fasting protocols in populations indicative of metabolic syndrome and those under undue chronic stress. This is something that would be best served as a short-term strategy in the leaner populations.[253,254]

Excessive periods of fasting and caloric restriction will increase the level of cortisol, raise blood sugar (caused by the cortisol dysregulation), and negatively impact thyroid metabolism and the support of androgens. In the case of the overweight or metabolically challenged individual, a manageable and sustainable meal structure lends itself better to the resetting of the hormonal axis and focusing on simple caloric restriction brought about by regulation of intake.

This, alongside an increase in output, is sufficient to initiate fat loss in the early stages. This, coupled with a reduction in carbohydrate intake, appears to yield the most success. Athletic (competitive) and diabetic populations would need to further consider both meal frequency and carbohydrate intake due to their potential impact on both insulin levels and performance.

Due to the suggested higher level of insulin resistance brought about by adiposity, the insulin response to foods will be amplified in obese populations. The short-term omittance in the early stages of highly insulinogenic carbohydrates could be seen as beneficial.

I often use the two-door scenario to explain this. If I forced a room full of people to fast for 10–12 hours and gave them the two-door option one is full of all the hypothetical "dirty food" they would love to eat, the other full of the more nutritious stable energy foods which door would they choose?

If you are inclined toward door one, you are probably metabolically inflexible to some degree: if not on a biological level, certainly on a psychological level. Therefore, perhaps showing a degree of insulin resistance or simply the bell is ringing, much like Pavlov's dog. Your body relies on carbohydrates as its primary fuel source and regulator of blood glucose the options beyond this are inhibited.

You will more than likely find a high percentage of the Western population like this. This, therefore, rules out the benefit of many fasting protocols for now and points us toward higher meal frequency, moving toward decreased meal frequency over time. Once fasting conditions can be achieved, there is a high likelihood that the individual is developing more physiological and psychological exibility and control. This is often seen in conjunction with a decrease in overall adiposity. The leaner they get, the more flexibility they will typically acquire due to the metabolic efficiency increasing, cells becoming more sensitive, receptors becoming more receptive, and transporters becoming more efficient.

An effect of this is an increased ratio of LBM over fat mass and, in synchronicity, an increase in training output. The clearance of glucose and metabolism of lipids becomes much faster, insulin sensitivity becomes higher, and storage capacity becomes much more efficient.[255–257]

Another indicator of a degree of insulin resistance is that following a high-carbohydrate meal, you may feel tired, lethargic, and more than likely resonate toward further carbohydrate ingestion. The metabolic and cellular response is muted; therefore, glucose entering the cells is impaired and fails to respond to the normal actions of insulin not completely eradicated, as it is not purely an insulin-dependent action.

The inhibitory signals that would normally prevent the liver from producing more glucose are also somewhat slowed due to the liver's insulin resistance. This leads to elevated blood glucose, mediated by the liver, and compounds the fact that, for these populations, fasting will only lead to further blood sugar problems. The goal must be to not only increase insulin sensitivity, but also to inhibit glucose output from the liver.

Increased meal frequency encourages meal-induced insulin production alongside an increase in thyroid hormone secretion. Keeping the liver healthy plays an enormous role in this entire regulatory process. A client's current situation relevant to these two facts can often be ascertained by the correct series of questioning alongside a food log within an initial client assessment.

Provided we have adequate protein (which we will discuss later), the use of protein as fuel is minimum but still of concern, especially in dieting individuals. This is where we must start to understand both the chronic and acute effects of food substrates, restrictions, and excessive consumption.

Upon any initiator of physical or emotional stress, catecholamines such as adrenaline (epinephrine), noradrenaline (norepinephrine), and dopamine are released alongside the corticosteroid cortisol as a basic evolutionary survival response.

GLUCAGON

In conditions of low blood glucose or in a fasted state, the liver acts as a reservoir for glucose and fuel to help normalize these levels to avoid hypoglycemia. As noted previously, the normal level of blood glucose is 5 mmol/l and any level above this will result in an increase in the secretory rate of insulin and a subsequent decrease in glucagon. In levels below this, glucagon increases and becomes part of a catabolic process, enabling the body to supply this shortage of energy and stabilize blood glucose levels.

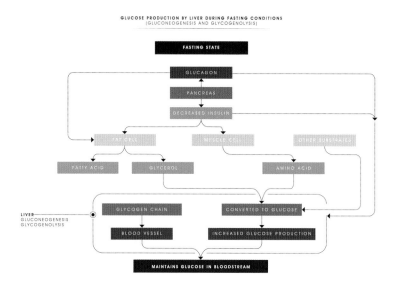

GLUCOSE PRODUCTION BY LIVER DURING FASTING CONDITIONS
(GLUCONEOGENESIS AND GLYCOGENOLYSIS)

Figure 15 Gluconeogenesis and glycogenolysis.

The liver does this through several pathways, the main ones being glycogenolysis, which converts glycogen into glucose, and gluconeogenesis, which allows glycogen to manufacture glucose from non-carbohydrate sources (such as amino acids), waste products (such as pyruvate, lactate, and glycerol), and fatty acids. Beyond this, the liver will then produce ketones from fats, known at ketogenesis. When the body acknowledges glycogen levels are low, it limits supply to ensure the organs that require sugar are fueled the brain, red blood cells, and kidneys. In doing so, ketones are formed and sugars are preserved.[165]

This is a catabolic process and reinforces, particularly in lean populations, why we cannot positively adapt tissue while simultaneously breaking down stored metabolites such as stored fat. Remember that in overweight populations, the degree of stored metabolites is higher, therefore favored in a better ratio over amino acids.

Our main priority during states of catabolism is largely therefore to preserve lean mass should physical development be the priority. The main initiator of glucagon secretion is a lowering of blood glucose. Glucagon and insulin together constantly strive to maintain glucose homeostasis. As insulin levels rise, glucagon levels lower and vice versa. As noted previously, alongside the elevation of insulin, there is the enzymatic release of LPL (which inhibits fat release). Glucagon, in contrast, releases the enzyme HSL (which liberates fatty acids).

The burning of fat as fuel therefore requires not only a hypocaloric state, but also a lowered level of insulin. Due to the inverse relationship that insulin and glucagon have, the presence of insulin will lower both glucagon and GH, both of which are necessary should we wish to tap into stored metabolites.

We can now understand the critical role of carbohydrates a little better. Carbohydrates have a protein-sparing effect, but also have the potential to keep insulin chronically elevated, serving to protect muscle tissue but inhibit the breakdown of fat. Insulin resistance, as mentioned previously, means that insulin in the blood never adequately lowers enough to enable the body to use glucagon, HSL, and therefore, its stored metabolic fuel.

Fat loss becomes almost impossible but the body will fervently protect lean mass. Improvement of insulin sensitivity and undertaking training that would increase glucose clearance would therefore help improve insulin sensitivity and the breakdown of stored metabolites.

In obese populations, the initial net lowering of carbohydrates and concurrent elevation of protein in a dietary strategy will improve insulin sensitivity, while the elevation of protein and dietary fat will stimulate glucagon release. As the compositional status improves, so does the management of insulin, glucose clearance, and thus the level and frequency of carbohydrate use. At this stage, protein to stabilize caloric intake will revert to a more stable maintenance level relative to the goals and metabolic requirements of the individual.

Due to its role, glucagon is classified as a catabolic hormone, breaking down larger molecules (metabolites) into usable energetic forms. This allows us to utilize fatty acids as energy. Insulin, in contrast, through the stimulation of glucose uptake, influences metabolism and anabolism.

THE THYROID

The thyroid reacts to stimuli brought about primarily by dietary intake. An increase in circulating thyroid hormones will cause a rise in thermogenesis and metabolic output, whereas a decrease slows both functions accordingly.[163]

These fluctuations, much like the actions of insulin and glucagon on blood glucose, help regulate the basal metabolism of the body. They also play a role in instigating breakdown of different substrates. The big player in most thyroid function is triiodothyronine (T3). This plays a role in nearly all of our physiological and metabolic actions.

Upon receiving stimuli, the hypothalamus releases TRH to signal the anterior pituitary to signal TSH. The follicles in the thyroid gland produce the two thyroid hormones T3 and its prohormone T4. Both are hydrophobic, so will diffuse into cells as opposed to needing a carrier.

When required, T3 and T4 are broken off the thyroglobulin into the bloodstream. The liver then directs the hormones to relevant tissue by releasing T4-binding globulin. When T4 reaches peripheral tissue, it must be de-iodinated by the protein 5 prime deiodinase, making the active version T3.

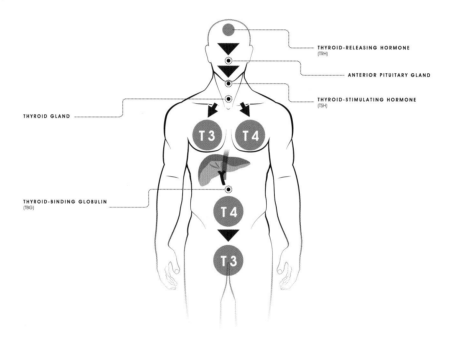

Figure 16 The thyroid gland.

When caloric intake is dropped, there is a significant reduction in thyroid hormone output. Part of this mechanism is that less T4 is converted to T3 and instead is converted to reverse T3 (RT3), as it is not needed due to the imposed metabolic demands. The RT3 contends for the same receptors as active T3, thus lowering metabolism accordingly and reducing proteolysis (breakdown of proteins into amino acids).[163,258]

More RT3 is produce when the body is under any type of emotional, physical, or biological stress, which can include fasting and sickness. Cortisol inhibits the conversion of T4 to T3 and thus causes increased production of RT3. The dilemma we have here is that in times of chronic, as opposed to acute, stress cortisol eventually lowers, also causing the same problem. Thyroid hormones stockpile in the blood and are converted to RT3 to contend with the high level of T4.

A few metabolic hormones, most notably testosterone and thyroid hormones, do not just use acutely produced versions in response to imposed demands. They are stored, depending on environment, as active or inactive forms. This is so they can be "released" when required. This is why dated medical tests are now redundant and paint us a clearer picture. Total testosterone and total T3 are fairly redundant without measuring the free or active versus inactive forms.

Loucks and Heath[258] found that when dietary intake in women fell below 50% of the normal dietary requirement, this adaptation occurred in as little as four days. Danforth et al., as long ago as 1979, also noted that both the caloric and carbohydrate content of the diet are important factors in thyroid metabolism.[259]

WHAT DOES THIS MEAN?

Underfeeding, fasting, or hypocaloric diets do appear to alter thermogenesis negatively if undertaken for more than a few days. Therefore, any such practice would be best served limited to only a few days if either an increase in lean tissue or reduction in body fat is the desired outcome.[188,260]

In contrast, overfeeding or hypercaloric diets[259] have been shown to alter the thyroid metabolism positively. Therefore, it would be safe to say that when caloric levels are substantially increased, it serves to support normal or increased thyroid metabolism. This appears to also be supported by the fact that the macronutrients play a role, particularly the inclusion of carbohydrate in the diet.

This would support the observation that, for many, during stages of dieting following the inclusion of a "cheat" meal or refeed, increasing both calories and carbohydrates has a positive metabolic influence. Most studies have been completed on "normal" weight volunteers. It would certainly be of interest to see the impact when studied around very lean individuals those that appear, in practice, to see the greatest response from inclusion of such cheat meals or refeeds.

We can look at this in many ways: one being as a metabolic "tortoise and hare" scenario.

- An acute, challenging, and unsustainable decrease in calories is followed periodically by a compensatory period in which calories are elevated and binging is encouraged (to some degree).
- A less acute, less challenging fluctuation or subtle wave between a hypo- .

and hypercaloric state that supports metabolic and endocrine hormones throughout mitigating the drastic psychological and behavioral changes required by the preceding situation.

Understanding the chronological history of your clients or your own dietary habits will help ascertain the caloric and carbohydrate levels required to support thyroid metabolism. Comprehensive blood work at this stage may also benefit those who can interpret it.

We could therefore assume that an overweight individual who has been on a consistently hypercaloric diet for long periods of time would show a good level of available T3. Perhaps however, the incidence of this is a little less than we would anticipate. The assumption that people are overweight simply due to consistently and chronically overeating would be shortsighted of us. The acute under- and overconsumption of calories at this stage seems to be far more apparent with the diet culture well in swing.

Sporadic patterns of hypo- and hypercaloric dieting initially create the adaptive responses that we have discussed. This slows metabolism accordingly, then ramps it up for extended periods of time to compensate for excessive caloric consumption. The evidence supports that we can do this, but the long-term (in excess of years) detriment of these patterns is yet to be studied or determined.[259]

A subtle wave between these states, in most cases, would be favorable to both well-being and metabolic health. However, one that hits strong peaks and valleys in a chronic and extreme fashion would be counterproductive.

If not, there is a likelihood that there is a binge pattern that may be indicated by a low level of T3 that was driven down by extended periods of VLCD with inadequate periodical time in an overfed state to bring it back to baseline. This would also implicate leptin, which would be responsible for the initial reduction in thyroid hormones. The action leptin would have on the hypothalamus would be to reduce TSH from the anterior pituitary, thus reducing overall secretion. Everything would be working together to simply adapt to a lowered caloric intake.

The classic 5:2 diet, in which people diet during the week at very low caloric levels then reward themselves on the weekends, will hold sway to such symptoms or issues in obese populations or those with dysfunctional behaviors and habits surrounding food. Coaches often encourage such an approach, as it expresses leniency and perhaps even kindness toward their clients. Again, we deal with an extreme scenario in which the imposed restrictions are so harsh even the coach sees them as such. The need to cheat is exacerbated by the extremes of restriction and once again, we implore the need to look at behaviors and habits in grave detail.

Considering this, the chronological dietary history may again yield some clues with those that have been on low-carbohydrate diets for extended periods. To elevate T3 back to its normal levels may be, in some cases a simple matter of increasing caloric intake alongside an elevation in carbohydrates. This, given that the thyroid is healthy, will influence directly and indirectly its secretion and activity. If the weight gain and dietary history were reflective of a high-carb diet, the cyclical lowering of carbohydrates would implicate better insulin sensitivity and maintain thyroid function by keeping carbohydrates routinely elevated. Something someone with such history would benefit from.

This, much like many other choices, leaves us with something that (given the consideration of history) helps us make decisions that manage themselves. A historically high-carbohydrate hypercaloric diet would require little to stimulate the thyroid, so a low-carb approach would be dominantly used until composition positively improved, alongside the desired level of insulin sensitivity. An approach using a ratio of both low-carb hypocaloric dieting to a higher, more than likely hypercaloric, level would yield a good state in which fat loss is supported while mitigating negative adaptations to the endocrine and metabolic hormones. As the individual became leaner, this ratio and reflective levels would increase.

One thing you can guarantee: in Western society, due to the abundance of food available, almost anyone on a restricted caloric plan will succumb, at some stage, to the body's energetic requirements. This, within the overly restrictive diet culture we find ourselves in, leads to binging, overeating, and the psychological implications we see that surround food. Compound this with the hormonal and largely endocrine changes and we are left with a metabolically challenged individual. The current support for flexible-style dieting is certainly warranted, but the application of it again remains questionable with the demographic that has followed the aforementioned patterns periodically. The goal ultimately is to lead people to a point of flexibility in choices with a somewhat automated control of intake and output.

LEPTIN

Leptin is an anorexigenic hormone that mediates energy expenditure, food intake, and therefore the overall levels of adiposity or fat mass.[260] This is done primarily through regulation of homeostasis, neuroendocrine function, metabolism, and immune function and is mediated by the CNS and peripheral tissues.[261] Anorexigenic hormones cause a loss of appetite, whereas orexigenic hormones stimulate it.

Carried through the bloodstream, leptin signals the hypothalamus to modulate caloric intake relative to energy expenditure, while balancing other physiological functions.[262,263] Leptin is part of the cytokine family and is synthesized primarily in the fat cells (adipocytes) and expressed by them.[190] It is an identified circulating factor in regulating the level of body fat in both human beings and rodents, supporting the notion that obesity is not merely brought about through poor dietary choices and lack of willpower but also compounding genetic and environmental factors.

We can also cross correlate this with the suggestion of the "set point:" the fact that people appear to display a regulated level of body fat that is maintained with this feedback loop. The mechanisms underlying why, once obesity levels are reached, there appears to be a resistance to fat loss are not fully understood. However, leptin certainly helps us understand some of the signaling pathways responsible.

When an individual loses body fat during longer periods of dieting, both the level of leptin and thyroid activity decrease. Correspondingly, a lower BMR is observed. Short term, this could be caused by, and related to, a reduction in insulin concentration. During periods of fasting, this reduction is rapid and acute and has been shown over periods of 24–72 hours.[191,192,264] This could be related to reduced insulin concentrations.

In response, through feedback mechanisms, hypothalamic modulators call for an increase in food intake that exceeds expenditure or a period of overeating. Similarly, an increase in adiposity would increase the plasma levels of leptin, resulting in a state of negative energy balance when food intake would be less than that of expenditure. In an ideal world, this would all self-regulate with the level of body fat corresponding to the level of leptin it elevates as obesity goes up, signaling adequate stored energy and the need not to eat.

Again, merely based upon observation with a hypothesized rationale, during rapid phases of fat loss, the adaptation or reversal of leptin resistance does not appear to run in synchronization. The levels of leptin therefore decrease in rapid succession with the overall fat mass. In using short-term and aggressive fat loss strategies, this leads to increased appetite and extreme hunger, as all the brain recognizes is the signal identifying a period of starvation.

Consider an individual on a plan that has a given short-term end point in which a coach can merely use willpower and the fact a client's motivation is currently high. This could be down to either accountability or, in some cases, the financial commitment the client has made. They are fundamentally on a countdown that will have elevated all of the hypothalamic and leptin-regulated modulators that signify overeating: NPY, MCH, galanin, orexin a and b, peptide YY, and andnoradrenaline.[260]

Now picture the signaling the brain is receiving alongside the psychological barriers many coaches have imposed on food what the client can and can't have or what is labeled "bad" or "good." Is it any wonder there is a binge mentality following extreme restriction and such a high failure rate?

The principle of specificity is quite simple. It implies that to improve at a particular Through what we know about leptin, we can deduce that the decrease of body fat cannot be a linear pursuit. Neither, therefore, can "weight loss" if it is to be supportive of long-term compositional improvements. It also supports the hypothesis that states of negative energy balance or catabolism cannot be maintained for long periods without satiety, hunger, compliance, and sustainability being questioned. As leptin is also stimulated by carbohydrate intake, it would also suggest that the omittance or reduction in carbohydrate intake long term would also negatively influence satiety signals.[144]

This would support that during periods of hypocaloric dieting, leptin levels would decrease and indications of hunger would increase. The inclusion of periodic refeeding would support rapid increases in plasma leptin, offsetting the likelihood of failure and poor dietary compliance.[265,266]

LEPTIN RESISTANCE

One of the major issues we have comparable to insulin resistance is leptin resistance. As leptin increases relative to the level of adiposity, it would be thought that the leptin would clearly indicate that there is adequate surplus energy to balance expenditure. What occurs with leptin resistance is the signal becomes muted. The brain cannot acknowledge that leptin is present; therefore, it continues to signal that the body is starving.[267,268]

In response to this, the brain continues to signal that the body is starving and therefore needs more calories. At the same time, it is signaling to simultaneously reduce energy expenditure. The more obese someone is, the steeper this curve becomes. Therefore, over time, as obesity levels climb, these signals become more and more muted, giving rise to stronger signals to overconsume.

Compound this with the complex psychological and behavioral adjustments, poor insulin sensitivity, and potentially dysfunctional thyroid hormones and you have a recipe for disaster. This is just the tip of the iceberg in going someway to understanding the mechanics of obesity. For our purposes, these are the major players and those we can positively affect.

At this stage, we need to question the endgame of flexibility in dieting. This does not mean reverting to the overly restrictive patterns that would implicate poor behavioral patterns and relationships with food. This means we must re-enforce better behavioral patterns and the inclusion of foods that are typically bracketed under the "clean" umbrella. Why? Simply because they satiate appetite better than less nutrient-dense options of the same macronutrient profile. "Good" and "bad" must always be replaced with "appropriate."

GHRELIN

Leptin and ghrelin share the same brain cells, so they regulate the satiety and hunger signals through a centralized effect. They are both, however, secreted in the peripheral aspects of the body. Ghrelin is primarily secreted by P/D1 cells, which line the stomach and help with production of the ghrelin antagonist leptin.[269]

Ghrelin, unlike the long-term regulatory effects of leptin, is a fast-acting hormone that appears to play a role in the initiation of eating. It is also inversely related to bodyweight. Ghrelin levels will elevate when weight loss is initiated and the stomach indicates it is empty. It signals the hypothalamus that there is a state of starvation or a shortage in energetic requirements; therefore, it becomes a physiological feeding initiator.[270–272]

Ghrelin's circulating levels decrease with feedings and increase before meals. The implications of ghrelin within a dietary strategy are largely useful as an indicator of satiety and the degree of sensation may help us with the prescription of caloric and meal frequency decisions.

At this stage, we probably do not know enough about ghrelin to conclude any positive dietary intervention. Its inverse relationship to leptin is more of a concern and assists in our understanding of it as an antagonist to those actions. I've found the work of Dostálová et al. to be helpful in understanding the current data we have on ghrelin and its actions.[271]

ANDROGENS

Androgens are the group of sex hormones often categorized exclusively as male hormones due to their impact on male morphological development. However, androgens are crucial for both male and female sexual and reproductive function, alongside their secondary sexual characteristics (such as body and facial hair and bone and muscular development).

To give you an idea of the impact of these hormones on human physiology and the aforementioned characteristics, it must be understood that men produce primarily androgens and women estrogens, but both sexes have a distinct and genetically determined maximal ratio of each.

Both androgen and estrogen activity are influenced by individual endocrine differences, ethnicity, phenotype, and individual health trajectories, alongside many other factors.

In men, the major androgen is testosterone. Men produce, on average, around 6–8 milligrams daily of testosterone. In women, the major androgens are

estosterone and the adrenal androgens. Women produce, on average, around 0.5 mg
of testosterone, 50% of which is produced directly in the ovaries and adrenal glands
and 50% of which is converted from the adrenal androgens. Adrenal androgens include
dehydroepiandrosterone (DHEA), DHEA-S, and androstenedione all of which are
weak steroid hormones or precursors.

When considering athletic and physique development, we must consider the ratios of
both androgens and estrogens. Our goal is to optimize the ratio through the limited
control we have over phenotype (environmental interactions, stressors, nutrition, etc.)
and an individual's health trajectory (the positive or negative rate of change against the
scale of age). Beyond that, without exogenous administration of such hormones, what
we can do is limited.

The body strives for balance: it likes to keep things such as hormones, muscle mass,
and bodyweight all within a narrow range or what we call homeostasis. This, over
long periods of chronic habitual change, can alter the aforementioned health trajectory I
spoke about and therefore these ranges vary. More often than not, this often leads to a
suboptimal androgen:estrogen ratio and a decline in overall health. Thus,
someone with a lowering of free testosterone will also experience a higher ratio of
estrogen. Someone, therefore, with an increase in estrogen will concurrently see a
decrease in testosterone.

Some of the effects of low testosterone (hypotestosteronism) and/or high estrogen
(hyperestrogenism):[274–286]

- Increase in depression
- Increased risk of diabetes (through what is largely seen as an increase
  of estrogen)
- Higher risk of prostate cancer
- Increased muscle loss
- Higher risk of heart and vascular disease
- Increase in fat deposition
- Lowered libido

Let's first look at the principal androgen testosterone and its production. This all
begins in the hypothalamus. The hypothalamus releases a hormone called GnRH that
then travels directly to the anterior pituitary, stimulating the release of LH. LH attaches
to the Leydig cells in the testes, signaling enzymes to convert cholesterol into
testosterone.

In women, androgens are produced in the ovaries, adrenal glands, and fat cells, with
their primary role being the production of estrogen. Therefore, estrogen becomes a
product of androgen metabolism.

In men, the apparent signs of an androgen imbalance are the increase in fatty tissue around the chest (gynecomastia) and the waist/hips. It will also be evident through an increase in ECF. In women, the virilizing and masculinizing effects are apparent in the same scenario.

FREE TESTOSTERONE DEFICIENCY

Any factor that increases SHBG will increase the amount of bound testosterone and lower the amount of circulating or "free" usable testosterone. Depending on the issue that lies with the individual, an excess or a deficiency in free testosterone would change how we would try to influence SHBG. Oral contraception or estrogen therapy, for women, would increase SHBG and lower free testosterone.

Long-term calorie restriction has been shown to lower serum total and free testosterone and increase SHBG independent of body fat.[287]

> *"To avoid this simple scenario, we must avoid chronic CR. Simply elevating above and below basal requirements ensures a dynamic balance with keeping testosterone and androgens at a healthy level while enabling us to keep body fat in control. This also has a concurrent impact on the thyroid hormones, which play a role in the synthesis of SHBG."*
>
> *~Rao[288]*

Zinc deficiency inhibits the enzyme aromatase, which converts testosterone into estrogen. You can lower this conversion by ensuring zinc blood levels are adequate. The more aromatase you have in your body, the more this conversion occurs.

ESTROGEN DOMINANCE

An increase in estrogenic stimulation can lead to excessive levels of circulating estrogen. Here are some of the most common factors:

- Excessive body fat As estrogen increases, so does fat deposition. Be cause fat cells make this hormone, this is a vicious cycle. The lowering of body fat will decrease estrogen.
- Insufficient progesterone Progesterone is used to make cortisol. Stress, the adrenals, and increased demand drag total progesterone levels down; thus, the dynamic balance the body requires between estrogen and progesterone is lost. This is the same with both men and women. An elevated estrogen balance will potentially increase ECF fluid, creating a softer and fuller look to the skin.
- Chronic exposure to estrogenoids and progestins These substances have an effect similar to estrogen and progesterone.

- Increase in aromatase Aromatase converts testosterone into estrogen. The adrenal hormone androstenedione will be converted into testosterone unless aromatase is present; in which case, it will be converted to estrogen alongside testosterone. Androgens have 19 carbons, whereas estrogen has only 18. Aromatase breaks off and attacks the 19th carbon, forming estrogen.
- Excessive alcohol intake In fact, any alcohol intake will have an impact. Alcohol depresses the CNS and lowers zinc, which is a fundamental requirement for efficient testosterone production.

SUMMARY

Decreasing stress to the adrenal glands will also decrease cortisol, which helps balance estrogen and progesterone. This applies to both physical and mental stress and is why you will often see that when people de-stress, they become leaner and vice versa. Chronic use of stimulants, CR, and general life stress can all contribute. It is very important to find a balance of recreation and work.

CHAPTER 14: CLOSING THOUGHTS

To think we can control or put a formula on a living organism and have a solid assurance of its response and outcome would be absurd. The very nature of our physiology and psychology in the ever-changing environment in which we live and breathe means the control we have, in the grand scheme of things, is minimal. What we do have are elements we can adapt and adjust according to an individual's responses and reactions. The mark of a good coach is someone who can note these subtle changes and act upon them.

The purpose behind this book was not to put a rigid formula or system around the pursuit of physiological change. It was intended to give you the reader insight into elements that play a large role, those we may influence, and those we have very little control over. There are the behaviors that we, as human beings, have developed throughout our lives. Environmental influences and the people around us inherently mold the way we perceive nutrients and foodstuffs.

Consider this with the knowledge we have already acquired and collectively achieved. This approach is in contrast to adducing evidence that might have instilled our belief in an authority. Nutritional dichotomies exist and we are surrounded by people who feel the need to belong to something and hold sway on a particular stance.

"Humans display the need to belong to something before the need to fully understand it."

~Phil Learney

Rather than making bold statements as to how it is, the thought process is rather, "How could it be?" Otherwise, we, much like those who have gone before, have failed to utilize our expertise and resources to guide someone effectively through each stage of change they require.

Science assists what we do and helps guide our practices. But, over time, scientific data is honed in light of new evidence and that evidence is often a reflection of coaches' resources and personal evaluations. As we come to the end of this book, I am once again privy to new information and studies that, was I able, I would gladly add. This will undoubtedly lead me to a second edition that includes newer research and further adapted plans, as information in this text is expanded upon or disproved based on this new research.

We must be able to embrace all that we have at our disposal. We must be able to take all popular programs and studies and be able to understand the intricacies behind them. Do they cater to the needs of the client in a positive light or as a means of compliance? Do they comply with the short-term purpose, yet offer little support for sustainability? Do they leave us with many questions to be answered? Do they offer very little support but stand true when compounded with understanding, rationale, and science?

We often falter with application. We have so much at our disposal with respect to methodology, much of which is often soundly and evidentially supported. The simple fact is the aforementioned need to belong to something overrides rationale and leads us to be biased. That inherent bias is what leads to misprescription and once again, the belief therein that what works for one must indeed work for all.

As always, we should be reflective and realize that what we know as coaches is merely scratching the surface of knowledge we can build upon and develop. The hope is that you can begin to understand through what this book has given you, alongside your current body of education that there is far more to consider with nutrition.

GLOSSARY OF ABBREVIATIONS

ACTH—adrenocorticotropic hormone

ADH—anti-diuretic hormone

ATGL—adipose triglyceride lipase

ATP—adenosine triphosphate

BMR—basal metabolic rate

cAMP—cyclic adenosine monophosphate

CNS—central nervous system

CNV—copy number variation

CR—calorie-restricted

CRH—corticotropin-releasing hormone

CSD—calorie-shifted diet

DHEA—dehydroepiandrosterone

DHEA-S—dehydroepiandrosterone sulfate

DPP IV—dipeptidyl peptidase IV

EAT—exercise activity thermogenesis

ECF—extracellular fluid

ENS—enteric nervous system

FFA—free fatty acids

FFM—fat-free mass

FSH—follicle-stimulating hormone

GH—growth hormone

GHIH—growth-hormone-inhibiting hormone

GHRH—growth-hormone-releasing hormone

GI—glycemic index

GIP—glucose-dependent insulinotropic peptide

GLP-1—glucagon-like peptide-1

GLUT-2/4—glucose transporter type two/four

GnRH—gonadotropin-releasing hormone

GSIS—glucose-sensitive insulin secretion

HBCD—highly branched cyclic dextrin

HCG—human chorionic gonadotropin

HDL—high-density lipoprotein

HSL—hormone-sensitive lipase

HTPA—hypothalamic–pituitary–adrenal

ICF—intracellular fluid

IGF-1—insulin-like growth factor 1

IFYM—if it fits your macros

LBM—lean body mass

LDL—low-density lipoprotein

LH—luteinizing hormone
LPL—lipoprotein lipase
MGL—monoacylglycerol lipase
MPS—maximal protein synthesis
MRUS—maximal rate of urea synthesis
mTOR—mammalian target of rapamycin
NEAT—non-exercise activity thermogenesis
NREE—non-resting energy expenditure
OCD—obsessive-compulsive disorder
OGTT—oral glucose tolerance test
PCOS—polycystic ovary syndrome
PDE3—phosphodiesterase 3
PI3K—phosphatidylinositol 3-kinase
PRF—prolactin-releasing factors
PSNS—parasympathetic nervous system
REE—resting energy expenditure
RMR—resting metabolic rate
RT3—reverse T3
SAID—specific adaptation to imposed demands
SHBG—sex hormone binding globulin
SNS—sympathetic nervous system
T3—triiodothyronine
T4—thyroxine
TBM—total body mass
TDEE—total daily energy expenditure
TRH—thyrotropin-releasing hormone
TSH—thyroid-stimulating hormone
VLCD—very-low-calorie diet

BIBLIOGRAPHY

[1]   Smith C. F., Williamson D. A., Bray G. A., and Ryan D. H. "Flexible vs. Rigid Dieting Strategies: Relationship with Adverse Behavioral Outcomes." Appetite 32, no. 3 (June 1999):295–305.

[2]   Westenhoefer J., Stunkard A. J., and Pudel V. "Validation of the Flexible and Rigid Control Dimensions of Dietary Restraint." International Journal of Eating Disorders 26, no. 1 (June 1999):53–64.

[3]   Kaye W. H., Bulik C. M., Thornton L., Barbarich N., and Masters K. "Price Foundation Collaborative Group: Comorbidity of Anxiety Disorders with Anorexia and Bulimia Nervosa." American Journal of Psychiatry 161 (2004):2215–2221.

[4]   Godart N. T., Flament M. F., Curt F., Perdereau F., Lang F., Venisse J. L., Halfon O., Bizouard P., Loas G., Corcos M., et al. "Anxiety Disorders in Subjects Seeking Treatment for Eating Disorders: A DSM-IV Controlled Study." Psychiatry Research 117 (2003):245–258.

[5]   Pollice C., Kaye W. H., Greeno C. G., and Weltzin T. E. "Relationship of Depression, Anxiety, and Obsessionality to State of Illness in Anorexia Nervosa." International Journal of Eating Disorders 21 (1997):367–376.

[6]   Fahy T. A., Osacar A., and Marks I. "History of Eating Disorders in Female Patients with Obsessive-Compulsive Disorder." International Journal of Eating Disorders 14 (1993):439–443.

[7]   Tanofsky-Kraff M., Ranzenhofer L. M., Yanovski S. Z., Schvey N. A., Faith M., Gustafson J., and Yanovski J. A. "Psychometric Properties of a New Questionnaire to Assess Eating in the Absence of Hunger in Children and Adolescents." Appetite 51 (2008):148–155.

[8]   Vannucci A., Tanofsky-Kraff M., Crosby R. D., Ranzenhofer L. M., Shomaker L. B., Field S. E., Mooreville M., Reina S. A., Kozlosky M., Yanovski S. Z., and Yanovski J. A. "Latent Profile Analysis to Determine the Typology of Disinhibited Eating Behaviors in Children and Adolescents." Journal of Consulting and Clinical Psychology 81 (2013):494–507.

[9]   Hebebrand J., Albayrak Ö., Adan R., Antel J., Dieguez C., de Jong J., Leng G., Menzies J., Mercer J. G., Murphy M., et al. "Eating Addiction, Rather Than Food Addiction, Better Captures Addictive-Like Eating Behavior." Neuroscience and Biobehavioral Reviews 47, (2014):295–306. DOI:10.1016/j.neubiorev.2014.08.016.

[10]   Bellisle F., Drewnowski A., Anderson G. H., Westerterp-Plantenga M., and Martin C. K. "Sweetness, Satiation, and Satiety." Journal of Nutrition 142 (2012):S1149–S1154.

[11]   Gearhardt A. N., White M. A., Masheb R. M., Morgan P. T., Crosby R. D., and Grilo C. M. "An Examination of the Food Addiction Construct in Obese Patients with Binge Eating Disorder." International Journal of Eating Disorders 45 (2012):657–663.

[12]   Gearhardt A. N., White M. A., Masheb R. M., and Grilo C. M. "An Examination of Food Addiction in a Racially Diverse Sample of Obese Patients with Binge Eating Disorder in Primary Care Settings." Comprehensive Psychiatry 54 (2013):500–505.
[13]   World Health Organization. Addiction.
[14]   Wilkinson R. G. and Marmot M. G. eds., Social Determinants of Health: The Solid Facts (Denmark: World Health Organization, 2003), 24–25.
[15]   Viner R. "Putting Stress in Life: Hans Selye and the Making of Stress Theory." Social Studies of Science 29, no. 3 (June 1999):391–410.
[16]   Ziegler D. R. and Herman J. P. "Neurocircuitry of Stress Integration: Anatomical Pathways Regulating the Hypothalamo-Pituitary-Adrenocortical Axis of the Rat." Integrative and Comparative Biology 42, no. 3 (2002):541–551.
[17]   Selye H. "Diseases of Adaptation." Wisconsin Medical Journal 49, no. 6 (1950):515–516.
[18]   Selye H. "A Syndrome Produced By Diverse Nocuous Agents." Nature 138 (1936):32.
[19]   Poesnecker G. E. "Selye Biologic Reaction to Stress Chart," in Chronic Fatigue Unmasked (Humanitarian Pub Co., 1999).
[20]   Wray C. J., Mammen J. M., and Hasselgren P. O. "Catabolic Response to Stress and Potential Benefits of Nutrition Support." Nutrition 18, no. 11–12 (Nov.–Dec. 2002):971–977.
[21]   Dallman M. F., Pecoraro N., Akana S. F., la Fleur S. E., Gomez F., Houshyar H., Bell M. E., Bhatnagar S., Laugero K. D., and Manalo S. "Chronic Stress and Obesity: A New View of 'Comfort Food'." Proceedings of the National Academy of Science of the United States of America 100, no. 20 (Sept. 2003).
[22]   Greenberg N. "Ethological Aspects of Stress in a Model Lizard, Anolis Carolinensis." Integrative and Comparative Biology 42, no. 3 (2002):526–540.
[23]   Vallès A., Martí O., García A., and Armario A. "Single Exposure to Stressors Causes Long-Lasting, Stress-Dependent Reduction of Food Intake in Rats." Regulatory, Integrative and Comparative Physiology 279, no. 3 (Sept. 2000).
[24]   Chagra S. "Effects of Chronic Stress on Neural Pathways Involved in Feeding." ETD Collection for University of Texas, El Paso (Jan. 2007) Paper AAI1449731.
[25]   Puhl R. M. and Schwartz M. B. "If You Are Good, You Can Have A Cookie: How Memories of Childhood Food Rules Link to Adult Eating Behaviors." Eating Behaviors 4 (2003):283–293.
[26]   Donche D. "FF Trainer Certification Guide." USA: Fatal Fitness.
[27]   "Training in Accordance to the 'SAID Principle'." TrainingforClimbing.com. (accessed Sept. 8, 2008).
[28]   Hubal M. J., Gordish-Dressman H., Thompson P. D., Price T. B., Hoffman E. P., Angelopoulos T. J., Gordon P. M., Moyna N. M., Pescatello L. S., Visich P. S., et al. "Variability in Muscle Size and Strength Gain After Unilateral Resistance Training."

Strength Gain After Unilateral Resistance Training." Medicine and Science in Sports and Exercise 37, no. 6 (June 2005):964–972.

[29]   Vertinsky P. "Physique as Destiny: William H. Sheldon, Barbara Honeyman Health and the Struggle for Hegemony in the Science of Somatotyping." Canadian Bulletin of Medical History 24, no. 2 (2007):291–316.

[30]   Sheldon W. H., Stevens S. S., and Tucker W. B. The Varieties of Human Physique (Oxford, England: Harper, 1940) xii, 347.

[31]   Mellin L. M., Irwin C. E., and Scully S. "Disordered Eating Characteristics in Girls: A Survey of Middle Class Children." Journal of the American Dietetic Association 92 (1992):851–853.

[32]   Bolonchuk W. W., Siders W. A., Lykken G. I., and Lukaski H. C. "Association of Dominant Somatotype of Men with Body Structure, Function During Exercise and Nutritional Assessment." American Journal of Human Biology 12, no. 2 (March 2000):167–180.

[33]   Ford E. B. Genetic Polymorphism (London: Faber & Faber, 1965).

[34]   Swallow D. M. "Genetics of Lactase Persistence and Lactose Intolerance." Annual Review of Genetics 37 (2003):197–219.

[35]   Ingram C. J., Mulcare C. A., Itan Y., Thomas M. G., and Swallow D. M. "Lactose Digestion and the Evolutionary Genetics of Lactase Persistence." Human Genetics 124, no. 6 (Jan. 2009):579–591.

[36]   Falchi M., El-Sayed Moustafa J. S., Takousis P., Pesce F., Bonnefond A., Andersson-Assarsson J. C., Sudmant P. H., Dorajoo R., Al-Shafai M. N., Bottolo L., et al. "Low Copy Number of the Salivary Amylase Gene Predisposes to Obesity." Nature Genetics 46, no. 5 (May 2014):492–497.

[37]   Novembre J., Pritchard J. K., and Coop G. "Adaptive Drool in the Gene Pool." Nature Genetics 39, no. 10 (Oct. 2007):1188–1190.

[38]   Mandel A. L. and Breslin P. A. "High Endogenous Salivary Amylase Activity is Associated with Improved Glycemic Homeostasis Following Starch Ingestion in Adults." Journal of Nutrition 142, no. 5 (May 2012):853–858.

[39]   Perry G. H., Dominy N. J., Claw K. G., Lee A. S., Fiegler H., Redon R., Werner J., Villanea F. A., Mountain J. L., Misra R., et al. "Diet and the Evolution of Human Amylase Gene Copy Number Variation." Nature Genetics 39, no. 10 (Oct. 2007):1256–1260.

[40]   Santos J. L., Saus E., Smalley S. V., Cataldo L. R., Alberti G., Parada J., Gratacòs M., and Estivill X. "Copy Number Polymorphism of the Salivary Amylase Gene: Implications in Human Nutrition Research." Journal of Nutrigenetics and Nutrigenomics 5, no. 3 (2012):117–131.

[41]   Bouchard C. and Tremblay A. J. "Genetic Influences on the Response of Body Fat and Fat Distribution to Positive and Negative Energy Balances in Human Identical Twins." Nutrition 127, no. 5 Suppl (May 1997):943S–947S.

[42]   Procino A. and Cillo C. "The HOX Genes Network in Metabolic Diseases." Department of Clinical and Experimental Medicine –

Federico II, University Medical School, Via Pansini 5, 80131, Naples, Italy.

[43] Karastergiou K., Fried S. K., Xie H., Lee M. J., Divoux A., Rosencrantz M. A., Chang R. J., and Smith S. R. "Distinct Developmental Signature of Human Abdominal and Gluteal Subcutaneous Adipose Tissue Depots." Journal of Clinical Endocrinology and Metabolism 98, no. 1 (2013):362–371.

[44] Gesta S., Blüher M., Yamamoto Y., Norris A. W., Berndt J., Kralisch S., Boucher J., Lewis C., and Kahn C. R. "Evidence for a Role of Developmental Genes in the Origin of Obesity and Body Fat Distribution." Proceedings of the National Academy of Science of the United States of America 103, no. 17 (2006):6676–6681.

[45] Deschamps J. and van Nes J. Development (Cambridge, U.K., 2005) 132, 2931–2942.

[46] Yu L., Gu S., Alappat S., Song Y., Yan M., Zhang X., Zhang G., Jiang Y., Zhang Z., Zhang Y., et al. Development (Cambridge, U.K., 2005) 132, 4397–4406.

[47] Campión J., Milagro F. I., Fernández D., and Martínez J. A. "Differential Gene Expression and Adiposity Reduction Induced by Ascorbic Acid Supplementation in a Cafeteria Model of Obesity." Journal of Physiology and Biochemistry 62, no. 2 (June 2006):71–80.

[48] Ford E. S., Giles W. H., and Dietz W. H. "Prevalence of Metabolic Syndrome Among U.S. Adults: Findings from the Third National Health and Nutrition Examination Survey." Journal of the American Medical Association 287, no. 3 (2002):356–359.

[49] Alberti K. G., Eckel R. H., Grundy S. M., Zimmet P. Z., Cleeman J. I., Donato K. A., Fruchart J. C., James W. P., Loria C. M., and Smith Jr. S. C. "Harmonizing the Metabolic Syndrome: A Joint Interim Statement." Circulation 120, no. 16 (2009):1640–1645.

[50] Rimm A. A., Hartz A. J., and Fischer M. E. "A Weight Shape Index for Assessing Risk of Disease In 44,820 Women." Journal of Clinical Epidemiology (1988).

[51] Stefan N., Kantartzis K., Machann J., et al. "Identification and Characterization of Metabolically Benign Obesity in Humans." Archives of Internal Medicine 168, no. 15 (2008):1609–1616. DOI:10.1001.

[52] Klein S., Fontana L., Young V. L., Coggan A. R., Kilo C., Patterson B. W., and Mohammed B. S. "Effect of Liposuction on Insulin Action and Risk Factors for Coronary Heart Disease." New England Journal of Medicine (June 2004).

[53] Baker M., Gaukrodger N., Mayosi B. M., Imrie H., Farrall M., Watkins H., Connell J. M., Avery P. J., and Keavney B. "Association Between Common Polymorphisms of the Proopiomelanocortin Gene and Body Fat Distribution: A Family Study." Diabetes 54 (2005):2492–2496.

[54] Sparrow D., Bosse R., and Rowe J. W. J. "The Influence of Age, Alcohol Consumption, and Body Build on Gonadal Function in Men." Journal of Clinical Endocrinology and Metabolism 51, no. 3.

[55]   Douchi T., Ijuin H., Nakamura S., Oki T., Yamamoto S., and Nagata Y. "Body Fat Distribution in Women with Polycystic Ovary Syndrome." Obstetrics and Gynecology (1995).

[56]   Mueller W. H. and Joos S. K. "Android (Centralized) Obesity and Somatotypes in Men: Association with Mesomorphy." Annals of Human Biology (1985).

[57]   Courtemanche C., Heutel G., and McAlvanah P. "Impatience, Incentives and Obesity." Economic Journal (2014). DOI:10.1111/ecoj.12124.

[58]   McEwen B. S. and Wingfield J. C. "The Concept of Allostasis in Biology and Biomedicine." Hormones and Behavior 43, no. 1 (2003):2–15. DOI:10.1016/S0018-506X(02)00024-7. ISSN 0018-506X.

[59]   Sterling P. and Eyer J. "Allostasis: A New Paradigm to Explain Arousal Pathology." in Fisher S. and Reason J. T. Handbook of Life Stress, Cognition, and Health (Chichester, NY: Wiley, 1988).

[60]   McEwen, B. S. "Protective and Damaging Effects of Stress Mediators." in Seminars in Medicine of the Beth Israel Deaconess Medical Center. New England Journal of Medicine 338 (1998):171–179. DOI:10.1056/NEJM199801153380307. PMID 9428819.

[61]   McEwen, B. S. "Stress, Adaptation, and Disease: Allostasis and Allostatic Load." Annals of New York Academy of Sciences 840 (1998):33–44. DOI:10.1111/j.1749-6632.1998.tb09546.x. PMID 9629234.

[62]   Schulkin J. Rethinking Homeostasis: Allostatic Regulation in Physiology and Pathophysiology. (Cambridge, MA: MIT Press, 2003).

[63]   Sterling P. "Principles of Allostasis." in Schulkin J. Allostasis, Homeostasis, and the Costs of Physiological Adaptation (New York, NY: Cambridge University Press, 2004).

[64]   Furness J. B. The Enteric Nervous System (John Wiley & Sons, 2008).

[65]   Rasmussen B. B. and Wolfe R. R. "Regulation of Fatty Acid Oxidation in Skeletal Muscle." Annual Reviews in Nutrition 19 (1999):463–484.

[66]   Havel R. J. and Goldfien A. "The Role of the Sympathetic Nervous System in the Metabolism of Free Fatty Acids." Journal of Lipid Research 1 (Oct. 1959):102–108.

[67]   Kalsner S., Frew R. D., and Smith G. M. "Mechanism of Methylxanthine Sensitization of Norepinephrine Responses in a Coronary Artery." American Journal of Physiology 228 (June 1975):1702–1707.

[68]   Mauriege P., Galitzky J., Berlan M., and Lafontan M. "Heterogeneous Distribution of Beta and Alpha-2 Adrenoceptor Binding Sites in Human Fat Cells from Various Fat Deposits: Functional Consequences." European Journal of Clinical Investigation 17, no. 2 (April 1987):156–165.

[69]   Dulloo A. G., Seydoux J., Girardierz L., Chantre P., and Vandermander J. "Green Tea and Thermogenesis: Interactions Between Catechin-

Polyphenols, Caffeine and Sympathetic Activity." International Journal of Obesity 24 (2000):252–258.

[70]   Belza A., Toubro S., and Astrup A. "The Effect of Caffeine, Green Tea and Tyrosine on Thermogenesis and Energy Intake." European Journal of Clinical Nutrition 63 (2009):57–64.

[71]   Griffiths R. R. and Woodson P. P. "Reinforcing Effects of Caffeine in Humans." Journal of Pharmacology and Experimental Therapeutics 246 (1988):21–29.

[72]   Kaplan H. I. and Sadock B. J., eds. Modern Synopsis of Comprehensive Textbook of Psychiatry 4th ed. (Baltimore: Williams and Wilkins, 1985) 4, 1106–1223.

[73]   Taylor R. L. "Design of the Nervous System." in Mind or Body, Distinguishing Psychological from Organic Disorders (New York: McGraw-Hill, 1982), 13–29.

[74]   Nurminen M. L., Niittynen L., Korpela R., and Vapaatalo H. "Coffee, Caffeine and Blood Pressure: A Critical Review." European Journal of Clinical Nutrition 53 (1999):831–839.

[75]   Griffin Jr. J. B. "Psychological Disturbances of Vegetative Function." in Walker H. K., Hall W. D., and Hurst J. W., eds. Clinical Methods: The History, Physical, and Laboratory Examinations 3rd ed. (Boston: Butterworths, 1990), Ch. 205.

[76]   Weir J., Noakes T. D., Myburgh K., and Adams B. "A High Carbohydrate Diet Negates the Metabolic Effects of Caffeine During Exercise." Medicine and Science in Sports and Exercise 19, no. 2 (1987):100–105.

[77]   Nehlig A., Daval J. L., and Debry G. "Caffeine and the Central Nervous System: Mechanisms of Action, Biochemical, Metabolic and Psychostimulant Effects." Brain Research Reviews (1992).

[78]   Astrup A., Lundsgaard C., Madsen J., and Christensen N. J. "Enhanced Thermogenic Responsiveness During Chronic Ephedrine Treatment in Man." American Journal of Clinical Nutrition 42, no. 1 (July 1985).

[79]   Hausman D. B., DiGirolamo M., Bartness T. J., Hausman G. J., and Martin R. J. "The Biology of White Adipocyte Proliferation." Obesity Reviews 2, no. 4 (Nov. 2001):239–254.

[80]   Spalding K. L., Arner E., Westermark P. O., Bernard S., Buchholz B. A., Bergmann O., Blomqvist L., Hoffstedt J., Näslund E., Britton T., et al. "Dynamics of Fat Cell Turnover in Humans." Nature 453, no. 7196 (June 2008):783–787. DOI:10.1038/nature06902.

[81]   Dreon D. M., Frey-Hewitt B., Ellsworth N., Williams P. T., Terry R. B., and Wood P. D. "Dietary Fat: Carbohydrate Ratio and Obesity in Middle-Aged Men." American Journal of Clinical Nutrition 47, no. 6 (1988):995–1000.

[82]   Kant A. K., Schatzkin A., Graubard B. I., and Ballard-Barbach R. "Frequency of Eating Occasions and Weight Change in the NHANES I

Epidemiologic Follow-Up Study." International Journal of Obesity and Related Metabolic Disorders 19, no. 7 (1995):468–474.

[83]   Bouton M. E. Learning and Behavior: A Contemporary Synthesis (Sunderland, MA: Sinauer, 2007).

[84]   Swinburn B. and Egger G. "The Runaway Weight Gain Train: Too Many Accelerators, Not Enough Brakes." BMJ 329, no. 7468 (Sept. 2004):736–739.

[85]   Ferraro R., Boyce V. L., Swinburn B., De Gregorio M., and Ravussin E. "Energy Cost of Physical Activity on a Metabolic Ward in Relationship to Obesity." American Journal of Clinical Nutrition 53 (1991):1368–1371.

[86]   Prentice A. M., Black A. E., Coward W. A., and Cole T. J. "Energy Expenditure in Overweight and Obese Adults in Affluent Societies: An Analysis of 319 Doubly-Labeled Water Measurements." European Journal of Clinical Nutrition 50 (1996):93–97.

[87]   World Health Organization. "Obesity: Preventing and Managing the Global Epidemic." WHO Technical Report Series 894 (Geneva: World Health Organization, 2000).

[88]   Visscher T. L. and Seidell J. C. "The Public Health Impact of Obesity." Annual Review of Public Health 22 (2001):355–375.

[89]   Mommsen S. and Foldspang A. "Body Mass Index and Adult Female Urinary Incontinence." World Journal of Urology 12 (1994):319–322.

[90]   Wardle J. "Aetiology of Obesity VII: Psychological Factors." in Force BNFT, Obesity. (Oxford: Blackwell Science, 1999), 83–91.

[91]   Swinburn B. and Egger G. "Preventive Strategies Against Weight Gain and Obesity." Obesity Reviews 3 (2002):289–301.

[92]   Stunkard A. J. "Socioeconomic Status and Obesity." In Cadwick D. J. and Cardew G., eds. The Origins and Consequences of Obesity. (Chichester: Wiley, 1996), 174–193.

[93]   Reidpath D., Burns C., Garrard J., Mahoney M., and Townsend M. "An Ecological Study of the Relationship Between Social and Environmental Determinants of Obesity." Health Place 8 (2002):141–145.

[94]   Bjorntorp P. and Rosmond R. "Neuroendocrine Abnormalities in Visceral Obesity." International Journal of Obesity and Related Metabolic Disorders 24, no. 2 Suppl (2000):S80–S85.

[95]   Summerbell C. D., Moody R. C., Shanks J., Stock M. J., and Geissler C. "Relationship Between Feeding Pattern and Body Mass Index in 220 Free-Living People in Four Age Groups." European Journal of Clinical Nutrition 50, no. 8 (1996):513–519.

[96]   La Bounty P. M., Campbell B. I., Wilson J., Galvan E., Berardi J., Kleiner S. M., Kreider R. B., Stout J. R., Ziegenfuss T., Spano M., Smith A., and Antonio J. "International Society of Sports Nutrition Position Stand: Meal Frequency." Journal of the International Society of Sports Nutrition 8 (2011):4. DOI:10.1186/1550-2783-8-4

[97]   Bellisle F., McDevitt R., and Prentice A. M. "Meal Frequency and Energy Balance." British Journal of Nutrition 77, no. 1 Suppl (April 1997):S57–S70.

[98]   Verboeket-van de Venne W. P. and Westerterp K. R. "Influence of the Feeding Frequency on Nutrient Utilization in Man: Consequences for Energy Metabolism." European Journal of Clinical Nutrition 45(1991):161–169.

[99]   Taylor M. A. and Garrow J. S. "Compared with Nibbling, Neither Gorging Nor a Morning Fast Affect Short-Term Energy Balance in Obese Patients in a Chamber Calorimeter." International Journal of Obesity and Related Metabolic Disorders 25 (2001):519–528.

[100]   Munsters M. J. and Saris W. H. "Effects of Meal Frequency on Metabolic Profiles and Substrate Partitioning in Lean Healthy Males." PLoS One (2012).

[101]   Garrow J. S., Durrant M., Blaza S., Wilkins D., Royston P., and Sunkin S. "The Effect of Meal Frequency and Protein Concentration on the Composition of the Weight Lost By Obese Subjects." British Journal of Nutrition 45, no. 1 (1981):5–15.

[102]   Jenkins D. J., Ocana A., Jenkins A. L., Wolever T. M., Vuksan V., Katzman L., Hollands M., Greenberg G., Corey P., and Patten R. "Metabolic Advantages of Spreading the Nutrient Load: Effects of Increased Meal Frequency in Non-Insulin-Dependent Diabetes." American Journal of Clinical Nutrition 55, no. 2 (Feb. 1992): 461–467.

[103]   Jenkins D. J. A., Wolever T. M. S., Vuksan V., Brighenti F., Cunnane S. C., Rao A. V., Jenkins A. L., Buckley G., Patten R., Singer W., et al. "Nibbling versus Gorging: Metabolic Advantages of Increased Meal Frequency." New England Journal of Medicine 321 (1989):929–934.

[104]   Leidy H. J. and Campbell W. W. "The Effect of Eating Frequency on Appetite Control and Food Intake: Brief Synopsis of Controlled Feeding Studies." Journal of Nutrition 141 (2011):154–157.

[105]   Chapelot D. "The Role of Snacking in Energy Balance: A Biobehavioral Approach." Journal of Nutrition 141 (2011):158–162.

[106]   Palmer M. A., Capra S., and Baines S. K. "Association Between Eating Frequency, Weight, and Health." Nutrition Reviews 67 (2009):379–390.

[107]   Solomon T. P., Chambers E. S., Jeukendrup A. E., Toogood A. A., and Blannin A. K. "The Effect of Feeding Frequency on Insulin and Ghrelin Responses in Human Subjects. British Journal of Nutrition 100 (2008):810–819.

[108]   Pearcey S. M. and de Castro J. M. "Food Intake and Meal Patterns of Weight-Stable and Weight-Gaining Persons." American Journal of Clinical Nutrition (2002).

[109]   Fabry P., Hejl Z., Fodor J., Braun T., and Zvolankova K. "The Frequency of Meals: Its Relation to Overweight, Hypercholesterolaemia, and Decreased Glucose-Tolerance." Lancet 2, no. 7360 (1964):614–615.

[110]   Cruz-Jentoft A. J., Baeyens J. P., Bauer J. M., Boirie Y., Cederholm T., et al. "Sarcopenia: European Consensus on Definition and Diagnosis: Report of the European Working Group on Sarcopenia in Older People." Age Ageing 39 (2010):412–423.

[111]   Pennings B., Boirie Y., Senden J. M., Gijsen A. P., Kuipers H., et al. "Whey Protein Stimulates Postprandial Muscle Protein Accretion More Effectively Than Do C Asein and Casein Hydrolysate in Older Men." American Journal of Clinical Nutrition 93 (2011):997–1005.

[112]   Nair K. S., Halliday D., and Griggs R. C. "Leucine Incorporation Into Mixed Skeletal Muscle Protein in Humans." American Journal of Physiology 254 (1988): E208–E213.

[113]   Stote K. S., Baer D. J., Spears K., Paul D. R., Harris G. K., Rumpler W. V., Strycula P., Najjar S. S., Ferrucci L., Ingram D. K., et al. "A Controlled Trial of Reduced Meal Frequency without Caloric Restriction in Healthy, Normal-Weight, Middle-Aged Adults." American Journal of Clinical Nutrition 85, no. 4 (2007):981–988.

[114]   Irwin M. I. and Feeley R. M. "Frequency and Size of Meals and Serum Lipids, Nitrogen and Mineral Retention, Fat Digestibility, and Urinary Thiamine and Riboflavin in Young Women." American Journal of Clinical Nutrition 20, no. 8 (1967):816–824.

[115]   Speechly D. P. and Buffenstein R. "Greater Appetite Control Associated with an Increased Frequency of Eating in Lean Males." Appetite 33, no. 39 (1999):285–297.

[116]   Pavlov, I. P. Conditional Reflexes (New York: Dover Publications, 1960).

[117]   Forbes G. B. "Body Fat Content Influences the Body Composition Response to Nutrition and Exercise." Annals of the New York Academy of Sciences 904 (2000): 359–365.

[118]   Wegner D. M., Schneider D. J., Carter S., and White T. "Paradoxical Effects of Thought Suppression." Journal of Personality and Social Psychology 53 (1987):5–13.

[119]   Wegner D. M., Shortt J. W., Blake A. W., and Page M. S. "The Suppression of Exciting Thoughts." Journal of Personality and Social Psychology 58 (1990):409–418.

[120]   Wegner D. M. and Zanakos S. "Chronic Thought Suppression." Journal of Personality 62 (1994):615–640.

[121]   Goris A. H. C. and Westerterp K. R. "Underreporting of Habitual Food Explained By Undereating in Motivated Lean Women." Journal of Nutrition 129 (1999):878–882.

[122]   Eston R. G., Shephard S., Kreitzman S., Coxon A., Brodie D. A., Lamb K. L., and Baltzopoulos V. "Effect of Very Low Calorie Diet on Body Composition and Exercise Response in Sedentary Women." European Journal of Applied Physiology 65 (1992):452–458.

[123]   Bandini L. G., Schoeller D. A., Cyr H. N., and Dietz W. H. "Validity of Reported Energy Intake in Obese and Nonobese Adolescents." American Journal of Clinical Nutrition 52 (1990):421–425.

[124]   Schoeller D. A. "How Accurate Is Self-Reported Dietary Energy Intake?" Nutrition Reviews 48 (1990):373–379.

[125]   Schoeller D. A., Bandini L. G., and Dietz W. H. "Inaccuracies in Self-Reported Intake Identified By Comparison with the Doubly Labeled Water Method." Canadian Journal of Physiology and Pharmacology 68 (1990):941–949.

[126]   Voss S., Kroke A., Klipstein-Grobusch K., and Boeing H. "Is Macronutrient Composition of Dietary Intake Data Affected By Underreporting? Results from the EPIC-Potsdam Study." European Journal of Clinical Nutrition 52 (1998):119–126.

[127]   Hotamisligil G. S., Shargill N. S., and Spiegelman B. M. "Adipose Expression of Tumor Necrosis Factor-A: Direct Role in Obesity-Linked Insulin Resistance." Science 259 (1993):87–91.

[128]   Feinstein R., Kanety H., Papa M. Z., Lunenfeld B., and Karasik A. "Tumor Necrosis Factor-A Suppresses Insulin-Induced Tyrosine Phosphorylation of Insulin Receptor and Its Substrates." Journal of Biological Chemistry 268 (1993):26055–26058.

[129]   Shoelson S. E., Lee J., and Goldfine A. B. "Inflammation and Insulin Resistance." Journal of Clinical Investigation 116, no. 7 (July 2006):1793–1801.

[130]   Kanai H., Sakamoto K., and Haeno M. "Electrical Measurement of Fluid Distribution in Human Legs: Estimation of Extra- and Intra-Cellular Fluid Volume." Journal of Microwave Power 18, no. 3(1983):233–243.

[131]   Rosenbaum M. and Leibel R. L. "Adaptive Thermogenesis in Humans." International Journal of Obesity 34, no. 1 (Oct. 2010):S47–S55. DOI:10.1038/ijo.2010.184.

[132]   Ray G. A. "Genetics Hypothesis of Nutrient Partitioning." Progress in Obesity Research 7 (1996):43–48.

[133]   Martinez. J. A. "Body-Weight Regulation: Causes of Obesity." Department of Physiology and Nutrition, University of Navarra, 31008 Pamplona, Spain.

[134]   Chaston T. B., Dixon J. B., and O'Brien P. E. "Changes in Fat-Free Mass During Significant Weight Loss: A Systematic Review." International Journal of Obesity 31, no. 5 (2007):743–750. DOI:10.1038/sj.ijo.0803483.

[135]   Hall K. D. "What is the Required Energy Deficit per Unit Weight Loss?" International Journal of Obesity 32 (2007):573–576.

[136]   Garthe I., Raastad T., Refsnes P. E., Koivisto A., and Sundgot-Borgen J. "Effect of Two Different Weight-Loss Rates on Body Composition and Strength and Power-Related Performance in Elite Athletes." International Journal of Sport Nutrition and Exercise Metabolism 21 (2011):97–104.

[137]   Hall K. D. "Body Fat and Fat-Free Mass Inter-Relationships: Forbes's Theory Revisited." British Journal of Nutrition 97, no. 6 (2007):1059–1063.

[138]   Janssen I., Fortier A., Hudson R., and Ross R. "Effects of an Energy-Restrictive Diet with or without Exercise on Abdominal Fat, Intermuscular Fat, and Metabolic Risk Factors in Obese Women." Diabetes Care 25 (2002):431–438.

[139]   Janssen I. and Ross R. "Effects of Sex on the Change in Visceral, Subcutaneous Adipose Tissue and Skeletal Muscle in Response to Weight Loss." International Journal of Obesity and Related Metabolic Disorders 23 (1999):1035–1046.

[140]   Rice B., Janssen I., Hudson R., and Ross R. "Effects of Aerobic or Resistance Exercise and/or Diet on Glucose Tolerance and Plasma Insulin Levels in Obese Men." Diabetes Care 22 (1999):684–691.

[141]   Dulloo A. G. and Jacquet J. "Adaptive Reduction in Basal Metabolic Rate in Response to Food Deprivation in Humans: A Role for Feedback Signals from Fat Stores." American Journal of Clinical Nutrition 68 (1998):599–606.

[142]   Maclean P. S., Bergouignan A., Cornier M. A., and Jackman M. R. "Biology's Response to Dieting: The Impetus for Weight Regain." Regulatory, Integrative and Comparative Physiology 301 (2011):R581–R600.

[143]   MacLean P. S., Higgins J. A., Jackman M. R., Johnson G. C., Fleming-Elder B. K., Wyatt H. R., Melanson E. L., and Hill J. O. "Peripheral Metabolic Responses to Prolonged Weight Reduction That Promote Rapid, Efficient Regain in Obesity-Prone Rats." Regulatory, Integrative and Comparative Physiology 290 (2006):R1577–R1588.

[144]   Levine J. A. "Non-Exercise Activity Thermogenesis (NEAT)." Best Practice and Research Clinical Endocrinology and Metabolism 16 (2002):679–702.

[145]   Weigle D. S. "Contribution of Decreased Body Mass to Diminished Thermic Effect of Exercise in Reduced-Obese Men." International Journal of Obesity 12 (1988):567–578.

[146]   Weigle D. S. and Brunzell J. D. "Assessment of Energy Expenditure in Ambulatory Reduced-Obese Subjects By the Techniques of Weight Stabilization and Exogenous Weight Replacement." International Journal of Obesity 14, no. 1 Suppl (1990):69–77.

[147]   Doucet E., Imbeault P., St-Pierre S., Almeras N., Mauriege P., Despres J. P., Bouchard C., and Tremblay A. "Greater Than Predicted Decrease in Energy Expenditure During Exercise After Body Weight Loss in Obese Men." Clinical Science 105 (2003):89–95.

[148]   Doucet E., St-Pierre S., Almeras N., Despres J. P., Bouchard C., and Tremblay A. "Evidence for the Existence of Adaptive Thermogenesis During Weight Loss." British Journal of Nutrition 85 (2001):715–723.

[149]   Rosenbaum M., Hirsch J., Gallagher D. A., and Leibel R. L. "Long-Term Persistence of Adaptive Thermogenesis in Subjects Who Have Maintained a Reduced Body Weight." American Journal of Clinical Nutrition 88 (2008):906–912

[150]   Ravussin E., Burnand B., Schutz Y., and Jequier E. "Energy Expenditure Before and During Energy Restriction in Obese Patients." American Journal of Clinical Nutrition 41 (1985):753–759.

[151]   Leibel R. L., Rosenbaum M., and Hirsch J. "Changes in Energy Expenditure Resulting from Altered Body Weight." New England Journal of Medicine 332 (1995):621–628.

[152]   Asami D. K., McDonald R. B., Hagopian K., Horwitz B. A., Warman D., Hsiao A., Warden C., and Ramsey J. J. "Effect of Aging, Caloric Restriction, and Uncoupling Protein 3 (UCP3) on Mitochondrial Proton Leak in Mice." Experimental Gerontology 43 (2008):1069–1076.

[153]   Bevilacqua L., Ramsey J. J., Hagopian K., Weindruch R., and Harper M. E. "Effects of Short- and Medium-Term Calorie Restriction on Muscle Mitochondrial Proton Leak and Reactive Oxygen Species Production." Regulatory, Integrative and Comparative Physiology 286 (2004):E852–E861.

[154]   Bevilacqua L., Ramsey J. J., Hagopian K., Weindruch R., and Harper M. E. "Long-Term Caloric Restriction Increases UCP3 Content But Decreases Proton Leak and Reactive Oxygen Species Production in Rat Skeletal Muscle Mitochondria." American Journal of Physiology - Endocrinology and Metabolism 289 (2005):E429–E438.

[155]   Hagopian K., Harper M. E., Ram J. J., Humble S. J., Weindruch R., and Ramsey J. J. "Long-Term Calorie Restriction Reduces Proton Leak and Hydrogen Peroxide Production in Liver Mitochondria." American Journal of Physiology - Endocrinology and Metabolism 288 (2005):E674–E684.

[156]   Dugdale A. E. and Payne P. R. "Pattern of Lean and Fat Deposition in Adults." Nature 266 (1977):349–351.

[157]   Payne P. R. and Dugdale A. E. "Mechanisms for the Control of Body-Weight." Lancet 1 (1977):583–586.

[158]   Payne P. R. and Dugdale A. E. "A Model for the Prediction of Energy Balance and Body Weight." Annals of Human Biology 4 (1977):525–535.

[159]   Kreitzman S. N. "Factors Influencing Body Composition During Very-Low-Calorie Diets." American Journal of Clinical Nutrition. 56 (1992):217S–223S.

[160]   Hall K. D. "Body Fat and Fat-Free Mass Interrelationships." British Journal of Nutrition (June 2007) 97, no. 6:1059–1106.

[161]   Miles C. W., Wong N. P., Rumpler W. V., and Conway J. "Effect of Circadian Variation in Energy Expenditure, Within-Subject Variation and Weight Reduction on Thermic Effect of Food." European Journal of Clinical Nutrition 47 (1993):274–284.

[162]   Mäestu J., Eliakim A., Jürimäe J., Valter I., and Jürimäe T. "Anabolic and Catabolic Hormones and Energy Balance of the Male Bodybuilders During the Preparation for the Competition." Journal of Strength and Conditioning Research 24, no. 4 (April 2010):1074–1081.

[163]   Rossow L. M., Fukuda D. H., Fahs C. A., Loenneke J. P., and Stout J. R. "Natural Bodybuilding Competition Preparation and Recovery: A 12-Month Case Study." International Journal of Sports Physiology and Performance 8 (Feb. 2013):582–592.

[164]   Hagmar M., Berglund B., Brismar K., and Hirschberg A. L. "Body Composition and Endocrine Profile of Male Olympic Athletes Striving for Leanness." Clinical Journal of Sports Medicine 23 (2013):197–201.

[165]   Kim B. "Thyroid Hormone as a Determinant of Energy Expenditure and the Basal Metabolic Rate." Thyroid 18 (2008)18:141–144.

[166]   Fontana L., Klein S., Holloszy J. O., and Premachandra B. N. "Effect of Long-Term Calorie Restriction with Adequate Protein and Micronutrients on Thyroid Hormones." Journal of Clinical Endocrinology and Metabolism 91, no. 8 (2006):3232.

[167]   Witbracht M. G., Laugero K. D., Van Loan M. D., Adams S. H., and Keim N. L. "Performance on the Iowa Gambling Task Is Related to Magnitude of Weight Loss and Salivary Cortisol in a Diet-Induced Weight Loss Intervention in Overweight Women." Physiology and Behavior 106 (2012):291–297.

[168]   Tomiyama A. J., Mann T., Vinas D., Hunger J. M., Dejager J., and Taylor S. E. "Low Calorie Dieting Increases Cortisol." Psychosomatic Medicine 72, no. 4 (May 2010):357–364. DOI:10.1097/PSY.0b013e3181d9523c.

[169]   Welle S., Matthews D. E., Campbell R. G., and Nair K. S. "Stimulation of Protein Turnover By Carbohydrate Overfeeding in Men." American Journal of Physiology - Endocrinology and Metabolism 257, no. 3 (Sept. 1989):E413–E417.

[170]   Kelley D. E., Mintun M. A., Watkins S. C., et al. "The Effect of Non-Insulin-Dependent Diabetes Mellitus and Obesity on Glucose Transport and Phosphorylation in Skeletal Muscle." Journal of Clinical Investigation 97 (1996):2705–2713.

[171]   Kelley D. E. "Skeletal Muscle Fat Oxidation: Timing and Flexibility Are Everything." Journal of Clinical Investigation 115, no. 7 (July 2005):1699–1702. DOI:10.1172/JCI25758.

[172]   Kelley D. E. and Mandarino L. J. "Fuel Selection in Human Skeletal Muscle in Insulin Resistance: A Reexamination." Diabetes 49 (2000):677–683.

[173]   Weir G. C. and Bonner-Wei S. "Five Stages of Evolving Beta-Cell Dysfunction During Progression to Diabetes." Diabetes 53, no. 3 Suppl (Dec. 2004):S16–S21. DOI:10.2337/diabetes.53.suppl_3.S16.

[174]   Mari A. and Ferrannini E. "Beta-Cell Function Assessment From Modelling of Oral Tests: An Effective Approach." Diabetes, Obesity and Metabolism 10, no. 4 Suppl (Nov. 2008):77–87. DOI:10.1111/j.1463-1326.2008.00946.x.

[175]   Matsuda M. and DeFronzo R. A. "Insulin Sensitivity Indices Obtained from Oral Glucose Tolerance Testing: Comparison with the Euglycemic Insulin Clamp." Diabetes Care 22, no. 9 (Sept. 1999):1462–1470.

[176]   Ratzmann K. P., Knospe S., Heinke P., and Schulz B. "Relationship Between Body Fat Mass, Carbohydrate Tolerance and IRI Response During Glucose Infusion in Subjects with Early Diabetes." Acta Diabetologica Latina 16, no. 1 (Jan.–March 1979):67–75.

[177]   Boelsma E., Brink E. J., Stafleu A., and Hendriks H. F. "Measures of Postprandial Wellness After Single Intake of Two Protein-Carbohydrate Meals." Appetite 54, no. 3 (June 2010):456–64. DOI:10.1016/j.appet.2009.12.014.

[178]   Müller M. J., Bosy-Westphal A., and Heymsfield S. B. "Is There Evidence for a Set Point That Regulates Human Body Weight?" F1000 Medicine Reports 2 (Aug. 2010):59.

[179]   Hall K. D. and Heymsfield S. B. "Models Use Leptin and Calculus to Count Calories. Cell Metabolism 9 (2009):3–4. DOI:10.1016/j.cmet.2008.12.006.

[180]   Conn J. W. and Newburgh L. H. "The Glycemic Response to Isoglucogenic Quantities of Protein and Carbohydrate." Journal of Clinical Investigation 15 (1936):667–671.

[181]   Nuttall F. Q. and Gannon M. C. "Plasma Glucose and Insulin Response to Macronutrients in Nondiabetics and NIDDM Subjects." Diabetes Care 14 (1991):824–838.

[182]   Iglay H. B., et al. "Resistance Training and Dietary Protein: Effects on Glucose Tolerance and Contents of Skeletal Muscle Insulin Signaling Proteins in Older Persons." American Journal of Clinical Nutrition 85, no. 4 (April 2007): 1005–1013.

[183]   Dolezal B. A., et al. "Concurrent Resistance and Endurance Training Influence Basal Metabolic Rate in Nondieting Individuals." Journal of Applied Physiology 85, no. 2 (Aug. 1985):695–700.

[184]   Josse A. R., et al. "Body Composition and Strength Changes in Women with Milk and Resistance Exercise." Medicine and Science in Sports and Exercise 42, no. 6 (June 2010):1122–1130.

[185]   Davoodi S. H., et al. "Calorie Shifting Diet Versus Calorie Restriction Diet: A Comparative Clinical Trial Study." International Journal of Preventive Medicine 5, no. 4 (2014):447.

[186]   Douyon L. and Schteingart D. E. "Effect of Obesity and Starvation on Thyroid Hormone, Growth Hormone, and Cortisol Secretion." Endocrinology Metabolism Clinics of North America 31 (2002):173–189.

[187]   de Rosa G., et al. "Thyroid Function in Altered Nutritional State." Experimental and Clinical Endocrinology and Diabetes 82 (1983):173–177.

[188]   Danforth Jr. E., et al. "Dietary-Induced Alterations in Thyroid Hormone Metabolism During Overnutrition." Journal of Clinical Investigation 64, no. 5 (1979):1336–1347.

[189]   Friedl K. E., et al. "Endocrine Markers of Semistarvation in Healthy Lean Men in a Multistressor Environment." Journal of Applied Physiology 88 (2000):1820–1830.

190]   Chan J. L., Heist K., DePaoli A. M., Veldhuis J. D., and Mantzoros C. S. The Role of Falling Leptin Levels in the Neuroendocrine and Metabolic Adaptation o Short-Term Starvation in Healthy Men." Journal of Clinical Investigation. 111, no.) (May 2003):1409–1421. DOI:10.1172/JCI17490. PMC 154448. PMID 12727933.

191]   Kolaczynski J. W., Considine R. V., Ohannesian J., Marco C., Opentanova ., Nyce M. R., Myint M., and Caro J. F. "Responses of Leptin to Short-Term Fasting and Refeeding in Humans: A Link with Ketogenesis But Not Ketones Themselves." Diabetes 45, no. 11 (Nov. 1996):1511–1515. DOI:10.2337/diab.45.11.1511. PMID 3866554.

192]   Kolaczynski J. W., Ohannesian J. P., Considine R. V., Marco C. C., and Caro I. F. "Response of Leptin to Short-Term and Prolonged Overfeeding in Humans." Journal of Clinical Endocrinology Metabolism 81, no. 11 (Nov. 1996):4162–4165. DOI:10.1210/jc.81.11.4162. PMID 8923877

193]   Klein S., et al. "Leptin Production During Early Starvation in Lean and Obese Women." American Journal of Physiology - Endocrinology and Metabolism 278 2000):E280–E284.

194]   Marniemi J., Vuori I., Kinnunen V., Rahkila P., Vainikka M., and Peltonen P. Metabolic Changes Induced By Combined Prolonged Exercise and Low-Calorie ntake in Man." European Journal of Applied Physiology and Occupational Physiology 53, no. 2 (1984):121–127.

195]   Garrel D. R., Todd K. S., Pugeat M. M., and Calloway D. H. "Hormonal Changes in Normal Men Under Marginally Negative Energy Balance." American Journal of Clinical Nutrition 39, no. 6 (June 1984):930–936.

196]   Dulloo A. G. and Samec S. "Uncoupling Proteins: Their Roles in Adaptive Thermogenesis and Substrate Metabolism Reconsidered." British Journal of Nutrition 86 (2001):123–139.

197]   Houston M. E. Biochemistry Primer for Exercise Science. (Champaign IL, Human Kinetics, 2006).

198]   Rudman D., DiFulco T. J., Galambos J. T., Smith R. B., Salam A. A., and Warren W. D. "Maximal Rates of Excretion and Synthesis of Urea in Normal and Cirrhotic Subjects." Journal of Clinical Investigation 52 (1973):2241–2249.

199]   Helms E. R., Zinn C., Rowlands D. S., and Brown S. R. "A Systematic Review of Dietary Protein During Caloric Restriction in Resistance Trained Lean Athletes: A Case for Higher Intakes." International Journal of Sport Nutrition and Exercise Metabolism (2013).

200]   Bowtell J. L., Leese G. P., Smith K., Watt P. W., Nevill A., Rooyackers O., et al. "Modulation of Whole Body Protein Metabolism, During and After Exercise, By Variation of Dietary Protein." Journal of Applied Physiology 85 (1998):1744–1752.

201]   Friedman J. E. and Lemon P. W. "Effect of Chronic Endurance Exercise on Retention of Dietary Protein." International Journal of Sports Medicine 10, no. 10 1989):118–123.

[202]   Meredith C. N., Zackin M. J., Frontera W. R., and Evans W. J. "Dietary Protein Requirements and Body Protein Metabolism in Endurance-Trained Men." Journal of Applied Physiology 66 (1989):2850–2856.

[203]   Pannemans D. L., Halliday D., Westerterp K. R., and Kester A. D. "Effect of Variable Protein Intake on Whole Body Protein Turnover in Young Men and Women." American Journal of Clinical Nutrition 61 (1995):69–74.

[204]   Tarnopolsky M. A., MacDougall J. D., and Atkinson S. A. "Influence of Protein Intake and Training Status on Nitrogen Balance and Lean Body Mass." Journal of Applied Physiology 64 (1988):187–193.

[205]   Phillips S. M. and van Loon L. J. C. "Dietary Protein for Athletes: From Requirements to Optimum Adaptation." Journal of Sports Science 29, no. 6 (2011):647–654. DOI:10.1080/02640414.2011.619204.

[206]   Bryner R. W, Ullrich I. H., Sauers J., et al. "Effects of Resistance vs. Aerobic Training Combined with an 800 Calorie Liquid Diet on Lean Body Mass and Resting Metabolic Rate." Journal of the American College of Nutrition 18, no. 2 (1999): 115–121. http://www.jacn.org/content/18/2/115.long.

[207]   Phillips S. M. "Dietary Protein Requirements and Adaptive Advantages in Athletes." British Journal of Nutrition 108, no. 2 Suppl (2012):S158–S167. DOI:10.1017/S0007114512002516.

[208]   Westerterp-Plantenga M. S., Lemmens S. G., and Westerterp K. R. "Dietary Protein – Its Role in Satiety, Energetics, Weight Loss and Health." British Journal of Nutrition 108, no. 2 Suppl (2012):S105–S1012. DOI:10.1017/S0007114512002589.

[209]   Walberg J. L., Leidy M. K., Sturgill D. J., Hinkle D. E., Ritchey S. J., and Sebolt D. R. "Macronutrient Content of a Hypoenergy Diet Affects Nitrogen Retention and Muscle Function in Weight Lifters." International Journal of Sports Medicine 9 (1988):261–266.

[210]   Evans E. M., Mojtahedi M. C., Thorpe M. P., Valentine R. J., Kris-Etherton P. M., and Layman D. K. "Effects of Protein Intake and Gender on Body Composition Changes: A Randomized Clinical Weight Loss Trial." Nutrition and Metabolism 9, no. 1 (2012):55. DOI:10.1186/1743-7075-9-55.

[211]   Mero A. A., Huovinen H., Matintupa O., Hulmi J. J., Puurtinen R., Hohtari H., and Karila T. "Moderate Energy Restriction with High Protein Diet Results in Healthier Outcome in Women." Journal of International Society of Sports Nutrition 7 (2010):4.

[212]   Griggs R. C., Kingston W., Jozefowicz R. F., Herr B. E., Forbes G., and Halliday D. "Effect of Testosterone on Muscle Mass and Muscle Protein Synthesis." Journal of Applied Physiology 66, no. 1 (Jan. 1989):498–503.

[213]   Norton L. E. and Layman D. K. "Leucine Regulates Translation Initiation of Protein Synthesis in Skeletal Muscle After Exercise." Journal of Nutrition 136, no. 2 (Feb. 2006):533S–537S.

214]   Antonio J., Kalman D., Stout J. R., Greenwood M., Willoughby D. S., and Haff G. G., eds. Essentials of Sports Nutrition and Supplements (Humana Press, 2008) XVII, 691.

215]   Wahren J., Felig P., and Hagenfeldt L. "Physical Exercise and Fuel Homeostasis in Diabetes Mellitus." Diabetologia 14 (1978):213–222.

216]   Gerich J. "Glucose Counterregulation and Its Impact on Diabetes Mellitus." Diabetes 37 (1988):1608–1617.

217]   Rorsman P. and Braun M. "Regulation of Insulin Secretion in Human Pancreatic Islets." Annual Review of Physiology 75 (2013):155–179. DOI:10.1146/annurev-physiol-030212-183754.

218]   Henquin J. C., Ravier M. A., Nenquin M., Jonas J. C., and Gilon P. "Hierarchy of the Beta-Cell Signals Controlling Insulin Secretion." European Journal of Clinical Investigation 33 (2003):742–750. DOI:10.1046/j.1365-2362.2003.01207.x.

219]   Frayn K. N. Metabolic Regulation: A Human Perspective 2nd ed. (Oxford, UK: Blackwell Publishing 2003).

220]   Ørtenblad N., Westerblad H., and Nielsen J. "Muscle Glycogen Stores and Fatigue." Journal of Physiology 591 (2013):4405–4413. DOI:10.1113/jphysiol.2013.251629.

221]   Ahlborg B., Bergstrm J., Ekelund L. G., Hultman E., and Maschio G. "Human Muscle Glycogen Content and Capacity for Prolonged Exercise After Different Diets." Forvarsmedicin 3 (1967):85–99.

222]   Burke L. "Nutrition Strategies for the Marathon" Sports Medicine 37, no. 4 (2007):344-347. DOI:10.2165/00007256-200737040-00018.

223]   Fogelholm G., et al. "Carbohydrate Loading in Practice: High Muscle Glycogen Concentration Is Not Certain." British Journal of Sports Medicine 25, no. 1 (1991):41–44. DOI:10.1136/bjsm.25.1.41.

224]   Sherman W. M., Costill D. L., Fink W. J., and Miller J. M. "Effect of Exercise-Diet Manipulation on Muscle Glycogen and Its Subsequent Utilization During Performance. International Journal of Sports Medicine 2, no. 2 (May 1981):114–118.

225]   Siri-Tarino P. W., Sun Q., Hu F. B., and Krauss R. M. "Meta-Analysis of Prospective Cohort Studies Evaluating the Association of Saturated Fat with Cardiovascular Disease." American Journal of Clinical Nutrition (Jan. 2010).

226]   Dreon D. M., Fernstrom H. A., Campos H., Blanche P., Williams P. T., and Krauss R. M. "Change in Dietary Saturated Fat Intake Is Correlated with Change in Mass of Large Low-Density-Lipoprotein Particles in Men." American Journal of Clinical Nutrition 67, no. 5 (May 1998):828–836.

227]   Siri-Tarino P. W., Sun Q., Hu F. B., and Krauss R. M. "Saturated Fat, Carbohydrate, and Cardiovascular Disease." American Journal of Clinical Nutrition 91, no. 3 (March 2010):502–509.

228]   Gardner C. D., Fortmann S. P., and Krauss R. M. "Association of Small Low-Density Lipoprotein Particles with the Incidence of Coronary

Artery Disease in Men and Women." Journal of the American Medical Association 276, no. 11 (1996):875–881.

[229]   Campos H., Genest Jr. J. J., Blijlevens E., McNamara J. R., Jenner J. L., Ordovas J. M., Wilson P. W., and Schaefer E. J. "Low Density Lipoprotein Particle Size and Coronary Artery Disease." Arteriosclerosis, Thrombosis, and Vascular Biology 12 (1992):187–195.

[230]   Mensink R. P. and Katan M. B. "Effect of Dietary Fatty Acids on Serum Lipids and Lipoproteins. A Meta-Analysis of 27 Trials." Arteriosclerosis, Thrombosis, and Vascular Biology 12, no. 8 (Aug. 1992):911–919.

[231]   Mulrow P. J. and Forman B. H. "The Tissue Effects of Mineralocorticoids." American Journal of Medicine 53 (1972):561–572.

[232]   McKay L. I. and Cidlowski J. A. "Physiologic and Pharmacologic Effects of Corticosteroids." In Kufe D. W., Pollock R. E., Weichselbaum R. R., et al., eds. Holland-Frei Cancer Medicine 6th ed. (Hamilton ON: BC Decker, 2003).

[233]   Dorgan J. J. F., Judd J. J. T., Longcope C. C., Brown C. C., Schatzkin A. A., Clevidence B. B. A., Campbell W. W. S., Nair P. P. P., Franz C. C., Kahle L. L., et al "Effects of Dietary Fat and Fiber on Plasma and Urine Androgens and Estrogens in Men: A Controlled Feeding Study." American Journal of Clinical Nutrition 64 (1996):850–855.

[234]   Key T. T. J., Roe L. L., Thorogood M. M., Moore J. J. W., Clark G. G. M., and Wang D. D. Y. "Testosterone, Sex Hormone-Binding Globulin, Calculated Free Testosterone, and Oestradiol in Male Vegans and Omnivores." British Journal of Nutrition 64 (1990):111–119.

[235]   Hämäläinen E. E. K., Adlercreutz H. H., Puska P. P., and Pietinen P. P. "Decrease of Serum Total and Free Testosterone During a Low-Fat High-Fibre Diet." Journal of Steroid Biochemistry 18 (1983):369–370.

[236]   Meikle A. A. W., Stringham J. J. D., Woodward M. M. G., and McMurry M. M P. "Effects of a Fat-Containing Meal on Sex Hormones in Men." Metabolism, Clinical and Experimental 39 (1990):943–946.

[237]   Hill P., et al. "Diet and Urinary Steroids in Black and White North American Men and Black South African Men." Cancer Research (1979).

[238]   Wang C., et al. "Low-Fat High-Fiber Diet Decreased Serum and Urine Androgens in Men." Journal of Clinical Endocrinology and Metabolism (2005).

[239]   Reed M. J., Cheng R. W., Simmonds M., Richmond W., and James V. H. "Dietary Lipids: An Additional Regulator of Plasma Levels of Sex Hormone Binding Globulin." Journal of Clinical Endocrinology and Metabolism 64, no. 5 (1987):1083–1085.

[240]   Venkatraman J. T., Leddy J., and Pendergast D. "Dietary Fats and Immune Status in Athletes: Clinical Implications." Medicine and Science in Sports and Exercise 32, no. 7 Suppl (2000):S389–S3895.

[241]   Van Harmelen V., Reynisdottir S., Cianflone K., Degerman E., Hoffstedt J., Nilsell K., Sniderman A., and Arner P. "Mechanisms

nvolved in the Regulation of Free Fatty Acid Release From Isolated Human Fat Cells By Acylation-Stimulating Protein and Insulin." Journal of Biological 274, no. 26 June 1999):18243–18251.

242] Paquot N., Schneiter P., Jequier E., and Tappy L. "Effects of Glucocorticoids and Sympathomimetic Agents on Basal and Insulin-Stimulated Glucose Metabolism." Clinical Physiology 15, no. 3 (May 1995):231–240.

243] Polonsky K. S., Given B. D., Hirsch L. J., et al. "Abnormal Patterns of Insulin Secretion in Non-Insulin-Dependent Diabetes Mellitus." New England Journal of Medicine 318 (1988):1231–1239.

244] U.K. Prospective Diabetes Study Group. "U.K. Prospective Diabetes Study 6. Overview of 6 Years' Therapy of Type II Diabetes: A Progressive Disease." Diabetes 44 (1995):1249–1258.

245] Garber A. J. "Incretin Effects on β-Cell Function, Replication, and Mass: The Human Perspective." Diabetes Care 34, no. 2 Suppl (May 2011):S258–S263.

246] Reaven G. M. "Pathophysiology of Insulin Resistance in Human Disease." Physiological Review 75 (1995):473–486.

247] Westphal S. A., Gannon M. C., and Nuttall F. Q. "The Metabolic Response o Glucose Ingested with Various Amounts of Protein." American Journal of Clinical Nutrition 52 (1990):267–272.

248] Khan M. A., Gannon M. C., and Nuttall F. Q. "Glucose Appearance Rate Following Protein Ingestion in Normal Subjects." Journal of the American College of Nutrition 11 (1992):701–706.

249] Krezowski P. A., Nuttall F. Q., Gannon M. C., and Bartosh N. H. "The Effect of Protein Ingestion on the Metabolic Response to Oral Glucose in Normal ndividuals." American Journal of Clinical Nutrition 44 (1986):847–856.

250] Nuttall F. Q., Mooradian A. D., Gannon M. C., Billington C. J., and Krezowski P. A. "Effect of Protein Ingestion on the Glucose and Insulin Response to a Standardized Oral Glucose Load." Diabetes Care 7 (1984):465–470.

251] Gannon M. C., Damberg G., Gupta V., and Nuttall F. Q. "Ingested Protein Has Little Effect on Glucose Concentration or Rate of Glucose Appearance in People with Type 2 Diabetes." Journal of the American College of Nutrition 18, no. 07 (1999):546.

252] Noakes T., Volek J. S., and Phinney S. D. "Low-Carbohydrate Diets or Athletes: What Evidence?" British Journal of Sports Medicine (May 2014). DOI:10.1136/bjsports-2014-093824.

253] Khani S. and Tayek J. A. "Cortisol Increases Gluconeogenesis in Humans: ts Role in the Metabolic Syndrome." Clinical Science 101, no. 6 (Dec. 2001): 739–747.

254] Goodpaster B. H., He J., Watkins S., and Kelley D. E. "Skeletal Muscle Lipid Content and Insulin Resistance: Evidence for A Paradox in Endurance-Trained Athletes." Journal of Clinical Endocrinology and Metabolism 86, no. 12 2001):5755–5761.

[255]   Goodpaster B. H. and Kelley D. E. "Skeletal Muscle Triglyceride: Marker or Mediator of Obesity-Induced Insulin Resistance in Type 2 Diabetes Mellitus?" Current Diabetes Reports 2, no. 3 (2002):216–222.

[256]   Goodpaster B. H., Krishnaswami S., Resnick H., et al. "Association Between Regional Adipose Tissue Distribution and Both Type 2 Diabetes and Impaired Glucose Tolerance in Elderly Men and Women." Diabetes Care 26, no. 2 (2003):372–379.

[257]   Ramnanan C. J., Edgerton D. S., Kraft G., and Cherrington A. D. "Physiologic Action of Glucagon on Liver Glucose Metabolism." Diabetes, Obesity and Metabolism 13, no. 1 Suppl (Oct. 2011):118–125. DOI:10.1111/j.1463-1326.2011.01454.x.

[258]   Loucks A. B. and Heath E. M. "Induction of Low-T~ 3 Syndrome in Exercising Women Occurs at a Threshold of Energy Availability." American Journal of Physiology 266 (1994):R817–R817.

[259]   Spaulding S. W., et al. "Effect of Caloric Restriction and Dietary Composition of Serum T3 and Reverse T3 in Man. Journal of Clinical Endocrinology and Metabolism 42, no. 1 (Jan. 1976):197–200.

[260]   Friedman J. M. and Halaas J. L. "Leptin and the Regulation of Body Weight in Mammals Nature 395 (Oct. 1998):763–770 DOI:10.1038/27376.

[261]   Dalamaga M., et al. "Leptin at the Intersection of Neuroendocrinology and Metabolism: Current Evidence and Therapeutic Perspectives" Cell Metabolism 18, no. 1:29–42.

[262]   Schwartz M. W., Woods S. C., Porte Jr. D., Seeley R. J., and Baskin D. G. "Central Nervous System Control of Food Intake." Nature 404, no. 6778 (April 2000):661–671.

[263]   Margetic S., Gazzola C., Pegg G. G., and Hill R. A. "Leptin: A Review of Its Peripheral Actions and Interactions." International Journal of Obesity and Related Metabolic Disorders. 26, no. 1 (Nov. 2002):1407–1433.

[264]   Casanueva F. F., et al. "Serum Immunoreactive Leptin Concentrations in Patients with Anorexia Nervosa Before and After Partial Weight Recovery." Biochemical and Molecular Medicine 60 (1997):116–120.

[265]   Mantzoros C., et al. "Cerebrospinal Fluid Leptin in Anorexia Nervosa: Correlation with Nutritional Status and Potential Role in Resistance to Weight Gain." Journal of Clinical Endocrinology Metabolism 82:1845–1851.

[266]   Myers Jr. M. G., Heymsfield S. B., Haft C., Kahn B. B., Laughlin M., Leibel R. L., Tschöp M. H., Yanovski J. A., et al. "Defining Clinical Leptin Resistance - Challenges and Opportunities. Cell Metabolism 15, no. 2 (Feb. 2012):150–156. DOI:10.1016/j.cmet.2012.01.002.

[267]   Bado A., Levasseur S., Attoub S., Kermorgant S., Laigneau J. P., Bortoluzzi M. N., Moizo L., Lehy T., Guerre-Millo M., Le Marchand-Brustel Y., and Lewin M. J. "The Stomach is a Source of Leptin." Nature 394, no. 6695 (Aug. 1998):790–793. DOI:10.1038/29547. PMID 9723619.

268]   Klok M. D., Jakobsdottir S., and Drent M. L. "The Role of Leptin and Ghrelin in the Regulation of Food Intake and Body Weight in Humans: A Review." Obesity Reviews 8, no. 1 (Jan. 2007):21–34

269]   Cummings D. E., Weigle D. S., Frayo R. S., Breen P. A., Ma M. K., Dellinger E. P., and Purnell J. Q. "Plasma Ghrelin Levels After Diet-Induced Weight Loss or Gastric Bypass Surgery." New England Journal of Medicine 346 (2002):1623–1630.

270]   Münzberg H., Flier J. S., and Bjørbaek C. "Region-Specific Leptin Resistance within the Hypothalamus of Diet-Induced Obese Mice." Endocrinology 145, no. 11 (Nov. 2004):4880–4889.

271]   Dostálová I. and Haluzík M. "The Role of Ghrelin in the Regulation of Food Intake in Patients with Obesity and Anorexia Nervosa." Physiological Research 58, no. 2 (2009):159.

272]   Eskelinen S. I., Vahlberg T. J., et al. "Associations of Sex Hormone Concentrations with Health and Life Satisfaction in Elderly Men." Endocrine Practice 13, no. 7 (Nov.–Dec. 2007):743–749.

273]   Martinez-Jabaloyas J. M., et al. "Relationship Between the Saint Louis University ADAM Questionnaire and Sexual Hormonal Levels in a Male Outpatient Population Over 50 Years of Age." European Urology 52, no. 6 (Dec. 2007): 760–1767.

274]   Small M., MacRury S., et al. "Oestradiol Levels in Diabetic Men with and without a Previous Myocardial Infarction." QJM 64, no. 243 (July 1987):617–623.

275]   Sewdarsen M. et al. "The Low Plasma Testosterone Levels of Young Indian Infarct Survivors Are Not Due to a Primary Testicular Defect." Postgraduate Medical Journal 64, no. 750 (April 1988):264–266.

276]   Carruba G. "Estrogen and Prostate Cancer: An Eclipsed Truth in an Androgen-Dominated Scenario." Journal of Cellular Biochemistry 102, no. 4 (Nov. 2007):899–911.

277]   Stone N. N., Fair W. R., and Fishman J. "Estrogen Formation in Human Prostatic Tissue from Patients with and without Benign Prostatic Hyperplasia." Prostate 9, no. 4 (1986):311–318.

278]   Rodriguez-Tolrà J., Barreda J. T., del Rio L., di Gregorio S., and Miranda E. F. "Effects of Testosterone Treatment on Body Composition in Males with Testosterone Deficiency Syndrome." The Aging Male 16, no. 4 (2013):184–190.

279]   Saad F., Haider A., Doros G., and Traish A. "Long-Term Treatment of Hypogonadal Men with Testosterone Produces Substantial and Sustained Weight Loss." Obesity 21, no. 10 (2013):1975–1981.

280]   Snyder P. J., Peachey H., Hannoush P., Berlin J. A., Loh L., Lenrow D. A., Holmes J. H., Dlewati A., Santanna J., Rosen C. J., et al. "1999 Effect of Testosterone Treatment on Body Composition and Muscle Strength in Men Over 65 Years of Age." Journal of Clinical Endocrinology and Metabolism 84:2647–2653.

281]   Traish A. M. "Adverse Health Effects of Testosterone Deficiency (TD) in Men." Steroids (June 2014).

[282]   Nettleship J. E., Jones R. D., Channer K. S., and Jones T. H. "Testosterone and Coronary Artery Disease." Frontiers of Hormonal Research 37 (2009):91–107.

[283]   Rosano G. M., Sheiban I., Massaro R., Pagnotta P., Marazzi G., Vitale C., Mercuro G., Volterrani M., Aversa A., and Fini M. "Low Testosterone Levels Are Associated with Coronary Artery Disease in Male Patients with Angina." International Journal of Impotence Research 19, no. 2 (March–April 2007):176–182.

[284]   Singh R., Artaza J. N., Taylor W. E., et al. "Testosterone Inhibits Adipogenic Differentiation in 3T3-L1 Cells: Nuclear Translocation of Androgen Receptor Complex with Beta-Catenin and T-Cell Factor 4 May Bypass Canonical Wnt Signaling to Down-Regulate Adipogenic Transcription Factors." Endocrinology 147, no. 1 (Jan. 2006):141–154.

[285]   Cangemi R., Friedmann A. J., Holloszy J. O., and Fontana L. "Long-Term Effects of Calorie Restriction on Serum Sex-Hormone Concentrations in Men." Aging Cell 9, no. 2 (April 2010):236–242.

[286]   Thijjssen J. H. H. "Hormonal and Nonhormonal Factors Affecting Sex Hormone-Binding Globulin Levels in Blood." Annals of the New York Academy of Sciences 538 (1988):280–286.

[287]   Tan R. S. "Impact of Obesity on Hypogonadism in the Andropause." International Journal of Andrology 25, no. 4 (Aug. 2002):195–201.

[288]   Rao G. N. "Influence of Diet on Tumors of Hormonal Tissues." Progress in Clinical and Biological Research 394 (1996):41–56.

[289]   Landau R. L., Bergenstal D. M., Lugibihl K., and Kascht M. E. "The Metabolic Effects of Progesterone in Man." Journal of Clinical Endocrinology and Metabolism 15, no. 10 (1955):1194–1215.